Living Beyond
Your
Heart Attack

EUGENE B. MOZES M.D.

Living Beyond
Your
Heart Attack

PRENTICE-HALL, INC.
Englewood Cliffs, N.J.

To Mary and Jim Rose

Acknowledgments

I WISH to thank those who helped to mold this book into the form in which it appears. My literary agent, Scott Meredith, first suggested the subject and gave me constant encouragement. Monroe Stearns, of Prentice-Hall, Inc., took a personal interest in the work from the beginning, and made valuable suggestions for needed changes.

But the greatest debt I owe is to my secretary, Mrs. Marion Allensworth, who typed patiently and with forbearance the innumerable drafts and redrafts of each chapter and who, by her criticisms and suggestions that always added to clarity in presenting facts, and by helping to locate and arrange source material from the immense and extensive medical literature, performed the task of collaborator rather than that of secretary.

I also wish to thank Robert A. Bruce, M.D., Associate Professor of Medicine, University of Washington, and *Geriatrics* for their kind permission to reproduce three charts appearing in the book.

E. B. M.

Contents

PART II
Are You a Candidate for Heart Attack?

Heart Attack

1

The New Outlook

DR. ROBERT WARTENBERG, a physician and medical professor at one of our leading universities, recently wrote a very appropriate letter to one of his doctor friends who had just suffered a heart attack.

> Dear Hans:
>
> I beseech and entreat you to read and heed what is in this letter. You will lick your heart trouble as I licked mine. And here is how I did it.
>
> . . . Look at me. I had 2 attacks, in '46 and '52, but resumed my teaching, research, and practice. I wrote 2 books and a couple of dozen articles, went twice to Europe, was half a year guest professor in Freiburg, and talked around in Austria and Yugoslavia. When I returned here, I found myself retired, but was rehired and I continued my teaching as before. I dictate every single day not less than three hours, and put my running nose in many people's business all over the world.
>
> All the doctors who attended me say it is a remarkable performance. How have I achieved it? What advice can I give in the light of my experience to a comrade in trouble?

Since he was writing to a fellow physician, he did not have to go into details about the various medications. However, having been a patient himself, Dr. Wartenberg could tell his friend how these drugs had worked for him and how he had regulated the thousand and one details of his daily life. But his best advice is summed up in these three sentences:

Do not make any drastic changes in your life. Do not resign any post, etc. Continue as usual, but cut your work.

And at the end of the letter he adds graciously:

A great factor in licking my trouble has been my wife, Isa, and so will be your Tessa.

The letter was written exactly ten years after Dr. Wartenberg had suffered his first heart attack.

Is the inspiring example of Dr. Wartenberg an exception? Or did he achieve this remarkable result because, as a doctor, he knew exactly how to take care of himself? Far from it. As a matter of fact, you can achieve exactly the same, and perhaps even more remarkable, result as Dr. Wartenberg did.

Every year more than a million persons have heart attacks. The majority are middle-aged men past forty-five, for males outnumber females by nearly three to one. The obituaries are full of such phrases as "died unexpectedly," "died from a heart attack" or "coronary occlusion." Newspapers carry stories of unexpected deaths of men in prominent positions locally or nationally. No wonder the words "heart attack" have become associated in the public mind as synonymous with death.

But if a person does not die after a heart attack, he is fully convinced that he is living on borrowed time, that his active life is over and that he is fated to become a "heart cripple." His wife, relatives, and friends anxiously advise him to "take it easy," "slow down," and watch fearfully his every step.

It won't ease his mind for some hale and hearty man of his acquaintance to tell him about the heart attack he himself suffered many years before. He thinks that the reason his friend has recovered so completely is that his finances allowed him to spend half of each year in Florida, and that he had the best and most costly medical attention.

The very words "heart attack" sound terrifying for the victim himself and for his whole family. Yet such anxiety and constant preoccupation with the condition of his heart may sometimes invite a second and perhaps more serious heart attack.

You Don't Have to Quit

Most persons have the erroneous idea that the victim of a heart attack must curtail all his activities and become practically an invalid. Actually, prolonged inactivity can do a great deal of damage to the heart. The worst thing a middle-aged man can do, whether he has had a heart attack or not, is to give up all physical activity and, after a lifetime of strenuous work, to become wholly sedentary all at once.

Dr. Paul Dudley White, the heart specialist, and President Eisenhower's chief consultant, recently published a study that directly contradicts the popular belief that hard work damages the heart. Dr. White examined the health records of 355 Harvard alumni who had played on the football team between the years 1901 and 1930, and noted how these ex-athletes had fared in regard to heart attack up to the year 1955.

The most interesting of his findings was that those men who after graduation had quit doing exercise of any kind were far more prone to heart attack than those who had maintained at least some kind of light or moderate exercise. Physical activity had apparently served there as a protection against the later development of heart attack. The more vigorous the regimen these ex-athletes had pursued after college, the less likely they were to suffer a heart attack. Naturally, few middle-aged persons, even ex-athletes, continue a strenuous program of activity. Yet, interestingly, not a single one of these ex-football players who did continue such a program developed heart attack.

This does not mean that the only way you can avoid a heart attack is to do everything in middle-age that you did when you were young. Nothing is more harmful, or more ridiculous, than middle-aged persons, men or women, "cutting up" and trying to pretend, in appearance and behavior, that they are still young.

What you should do is taper off gradually, instead of retiring to the pleasures of the table. Act your age.

On the other side of the ledger are vigorous, over-ambitious, and over-active middle-aged men who, after a heart attack, are unwilling to make the slightest compromise. They drive themselves as hard as ever, thinking that they have little enough time left to accomplish what they have set out to do. Such an attitude is just as fatalistic as that of the man who is ready to curl up and wait patiently for death.

Modern medicine can do a good deal for the victim of a heart attack. Ultimately, however, *the success of any kind of treatment will depend on you.*

Even Dr. Wartenberg, a physician himself, who knew even the smallest medical details of his own disease, had to learn for himself what his symptoms actually meant and how to rearrange his life accordingly. How much more important it is for the average person to learn the basic facts concerning heart attack. For an intelligent understanding of all the facts involved in it will enable him to cooperate with his doctor toward his own recovery. But above all, by knowing what is going on in his heart, he will overcome the unreasonable fear that today is associated with heart attack.

Sudden Death Is Rare

To the average person, heart attack means sudden and almost inevitable death, with only a few persons lucky enough to survive more than a few hours or, at most, days. Actually, the facts are just the opposite. Statistics show that no more than 10 to 15 of every 100 persons who suffer a heart attack die immediately. Eighty-five to 90 per cent recover from it. The vast majority recover so completely that they are able to return to their former occupations with little or no disability.

One physician kept an accurate record for more than twenty years of 100 men and women who had suffered a heart attack. Sixty-six of these men and women were still alive and doing well after ten years. At the end of twenty years, 14 of them were still living and, for all purposes, in excellent health. Every one of these persons was past middle age when he suffered his heart attack.

The longest authenticated record of survival is the case of a man who suffered a heart attack at the age of forty and died at the age of eighty. An equally remarkable record is that of a man who suffered a heart attack when he was fifty and died thirty-six years later.

Your chances are far better than you imagined. The odds are very much in your favor.

Ability to Work

Until about twenty years ago, even physicians considered a person who had suffered a heart attack as totally and permanently disabled. He was practically forced to live the life of a heart cripple.

What a difference today! Now physicians agree that the great majority of persons who recover from the initial attack —and that, of course, includes President Eisenhower—will be able to resume light activities two to three months after the attack, and gradually increase the activity until they can return to their former full schedule.

Drs. Rosenbaum and Levine, for example, reported the fate of 345 patients who had survived a heart attack. Thirty per cent of them resumed full-time work, 45 per cent partial work, 22 per cent had to choose some other employment which required less exertion, *but only 3 per cent were totally incapacitated.*

Even insurance companies have radically changed their attitude toward heart attack victims. They no longer automatically reject the applicant as a totally uninsurable risk.

Recovery can be so complete that the heart function is practically the same as that of a person who never had a heart attack. Survivors have no symptoms whatever, do not tire easily, have no pain, and sometimes can even perform heavy manual labor.

How complete recovery can be is shown by a special study of persons in one city in Tennessee who had suffered heart attack and subsequently returned to their former occupations. For those who survived at least three years, the mortality rate was practically the same as for the general population of Tennessee of the same age, sex, and racial distribution.

What Is a Heart Attack?

Most persons who suffer a sudden heart attack are seemingly in the pink of health. They may even have had a thorough examination of the heart only a week or so before that showed not the slightest sign of heart trouble.

Then what, exactly, brings on the heart attack, like a bolt of lightning out of a clear sky? Most people think that the heart gives out because of overwork, worry, or something that gets into the blood and suddenly stops the heart's working. Actually, the conditions that ultimately led to the heart attack have been laid down over a good many years, and have built up gradually to a climax.

The main reason for misunderstanding, and the source of exaggerated fear of heart attack in the mind of the average person, is that he confuses heart attack with heart disease. *Heart disease has no connection whatever with heart attack.*

There are many kinds of heart diseases, but the most common one is of a mechanical nature. The chambers of the heart are separated by valves that open and close with each heart beat. These valves must open wide and easily, so that the blood can be pushed through the opening without the slightest difficulty. When they close, they must be closed so perfectly that not a drop trickles back in the wrong direction.

In the usual kind of heart disease, these valves do not function efficiently. Either they do not open wide enough or they do not close completely. The result is that the heart must work harder in order to make up for the constant deficit. The man who has this kind of heart trouble, naturally, knows all about it and, by taking care of his heart, he can live comfortably and can even work to whatever extent his doctors allow.

Most people think that heart attack is brought on because

a man has this kind of heart disease. Actually, what brings on a heart attack is not a heart disease of this kind at all. The heart of a person who suffers a heart attack may be in perfect mechanical condition. But there is something wrong with the artery of the heart itself, called the *coronary artery*.

The coronary artery has only one function, and that is to supply the heart with blood continually and without the slightest interruption. It is like a pipeline that carries blood to all parts of the heart. As long as this pipeline is open, even if it is somewhat rusted inside, the heart will receive enough blood to function in perfect order.

However, the minute one tiny branch of this intricate pipe system is shut down so completely that not a trickle of blood can get through to the particular small portion of the heart nourished by it, the heart as a whole suffers and the person is stricken by a heart attack. The heart muscle has suffered a slight wound.

If you wish to banish unnecessary fear, simply remember that after the supply system has been repaired, the heart is again practically as good as it ever was. The temporary interruption of its blood supply has not the slightest effect on the working of the valves of the heart. So far as mechanical arrangement is concerned, the person who has suffered a heart attack does *not* have heart disease in the usual sense of the word.

The Heart Is the Toughest Organ in the Body

The reason most people are so frightened at the words "heart attack" is that they believe the heart is an extremely delicate organ, that if the slightest thing goes wrong with it, it will stop working.

Actually, the heart is the toughest and strongest muscle in the body.

The amount of work the heart performs is almost unbelievable. The energy it puts forth in every twenty-four hours would be enough to carry a man weighing 150 pounds from street level to the top of a three-story building. The amount of energy it produces during a life span of three score years and ten would, if applied at once, be sufficient to lift the biggest battleship fourteen feet out of the water.

It is a powerful pump that never stops working even for a fraction of a second. It must supply blood to every cell in the body, constantly and without any interruption. To do this, the heart pumps through the blood vessels of the entire body five to ten tons of blood every twenty-four hours.

Unlike any machine made by man, it can adjust itself instantly and adequately to the ever-changing demands of the body. If you work, exercise, or perform any task, your muscles need more blood. The heart sees to it that more blood is rushed to the muscles you are using. For example, if you are at rest, the heart pumps into the blood vessels about five quarts of blood every minute. However, in a trained athlete, after extremely severe exercise the output per minute can amount to more than 38 quarts. After average exercise it is ten to fifteen quarts.

The capacity of the heart to respond smoothly and seemingly effortlessly to all demands of the body is known medically as the *cardiac reserve*. The cardiac reserve is many times greater than even the most exacting manual labor will ever call for. This heart reserve is the reason why the majority of persons can get safely through the first critical period after a heart attack.

The Damaged Heart

If you are doing moderate exercise, your heart may be working as much as six times harder than it does when you are in bed. This is the reason your doctor insists that you rest your heart immediately after a heart attack. He will also tell you how to avoid putting the least strain on a recently damaged heart.

But he will also insist that you should not be invalid too long. That little wound in the heart muscle *begins to heal almost from the moment you have sustained it*. After it has healed, your heart will contract better and better as the days, weeks, and months go by. If you are lucky, the fact that you had a heart attack will make no difference whatsoever in your heart's ability to work. In others, there will be some difference, but it will be only slight. In still others, of course, the after-effect will be somewhat more severe.

Until the healing is completed, there will be some limitation to your activity. However, the period of this severe limitation of activity must not be too long.

The year 1955 will probably turn out to have been the turning point in the treatment of heart attack. Until that time, physicians had prescribed six-week bed rest, lying flat on the back absolutely motionless, for every patient. In that year, two studies were published which proved that such regimen was not only unnecessary but may have been actually harmful in some cases.

After you leave the hospital, although the doctor has many ways to test the capacity of your heart at that stage, no one but you will be able to gauge accurately what you can and cannot do. You will be able to do this intelligently only if you thoroughly understand what is going on inside your heart, what the warning signs are that tell you to slow down temporarily. You must altogether arrange your life in such a way as to insure complete recovery. Complete recovery—and by complete recovery I actually mean that the person is every bit as good as he was before his heart attack—*is the rule rather than the exception.*

Sure enough, a heart attack is a serious incident. Its significance is not to be minimized. However, with the many highly effective new drugs, and a far better understanding by physicians of what is going on in the body when the heart has suffered a temporary breakdown, the outlook for the average patient is immeasurably better today than it was only a decade or so ago. You will recall the practically daily rounds of golf President Eisenhower plays in all weather, and how he performs the exacting duties of his office. His case is not an exceptional one.

"We now have seen," writes Dr. Arthur M. Master, one of the foremost authorities on heart attack, "scores of patients who have had no symptoms whatsoever for from two to twenty years after an acute coronary occlusion with infarction. They live completely normal lives, often work long hours and under tension, and occasionally even perform heavy manual work."

As one heart specialist remarked, it is a curious fact that most Americans, yes, even boys, know a good deal more about automobile engines than they do about their own motor apparatus. To this statement we may add that what they think they know is often highly erroneous. This incorrect information can do even more harm than no knowledge at all.

Although the finest points about the function of the heart are extraordinarily complex and complicated, the basic facts are easily comprehensible to everyone with average intelligence. You do not need to go through the rigorous courses of a medical education. But you do need a clear picture of what happens to the heart when it is struck down seemingly in the peak of health.

2

Your Coronary

The Heart Is a Pump

The body is composed of trillions and trillions of micro-scopic-sized building bricks, the cells. Each of these cells is a living organism in its own right and needs a constant and uninterrupted supply of fuel. The fuel in this case is the blood, with its content of all nourishing elements.

The blood is delivered to the cells through extraordinarily fine tubes, each incomparably thinner than the finest hair, 7 to 15 ten-thousandths of an inch in diameter. These fine tubes are called *capillaries*. The capillaries are the branches of somewhat larger tubes, called *arterioles* (diminutive arteries). These arterioles are themselves branches of still larger blood vessels, the *arteries*. The arteries stem from the main pipe line of the body, the *aorta*. The aorta itself comes out from the left chamber of the heart. So it is that the blood delivered from the heart through these subdivisions of ever finer tubes reaches its ultimate destination: the cells.

This system of distribution may be compared to the water supply of a house and its rooms. The heart is the reservoir or central plant, the aorta is the main, the arteries and arterioles are the water pipes going to each house. The capillaries may be thought of as even smaller pipes delivering water to the kitchen, basement, bathroom, and to every room that is provided with a branch.

But to understand the circulatory system properly, you need to know what happens after the blood has been delivered to the cells. The capillaries carry nourishing blood to every cell in the body. The cells, as they function, break down this nourishment, some of which will no longer be needed and has to be disposed of. This waste material is returned to the capillaries.

The capillaries, exactly like tributaries of a river, empty into the veins. These veins then empty into even larger veins, all of which in turn open into the two largest veins of the body. The used blood from the upper part of the body drains into one of these main collecting tubes, while that from the lower part of the body empties into the other one. Both of these empty into the right side of the heart.

In order to complete the entire picture of circulation, it should be added that the blood that is returned to the right side of the heart from the veins is sent first to the lungs where it picks up oxygen from the air. Then the blood, thus refreshed, is returned to the left side of the heart.

The body is honeycombed by an interconnected system of blood vessels, the function of which is to carry nourishment to the cells and to carry away from them what is no longer needed. If we could place end to end all these branches in the entire body, including the finest ones, they would stretch to one hundred thousand miles!

The driving power for this pumping is provided by the heart. With each contraction the heart squeezes some three ounces of blood into the aorta. Contractions occur at the rate of some 60 to 80 times every minute.

Like any other organ of the body, the heart itself needs a constant and uninterrupted supply of blood in order to function properly. This is delivered to the heart by the heart's own artery, called the *coronary artery*. Because the functioning of the heart depends entirely on regular delivery of its fuel supply through the coronary artery, it is obvious that the coronary artery is the most important artery in the entire body.

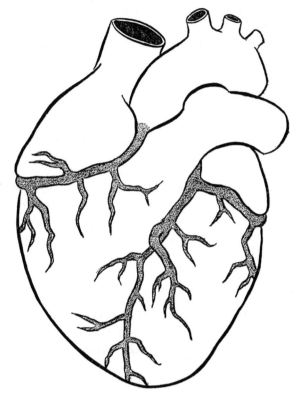

Figure 1. THE CORONARY ARTERY.

The Coronary Artery

The coronary artery is named from the Latin word for wreath, "corona," because its various branches cover the heart like a wreath. Actually, there are two coronary arteries, the right and the left. Both of these originate from the aorta and divide and subdivide into ever smaller branches until they reach every nook and corner of the heart, carrying blood to every cell of it.

When you want to speed up your car, you push down on the accelerator to get more gas. This is exactly what happens when the heart has to work harder. It needs more blood to increase its function. Therefore, the coronaries must deliver varying amounts of blood according to the momentary need of the heart.

How enormous such changes can be, may be judged by experiments performed on dogs. Investigators found that the coronary arteries of dogs while performing exercise on a treadmill delivered 400 per cent more blood per minute than when the animal was at rest. Even after a meal the flow increased about 84 per cent above that of the resting state. That is why doctors warn patients who are just recovering from a heart attack not to overwork their coronaries by eating too heavy a meal.

In order for the coronary arteries to perform their duties properly, the channels of these arteries, down to the smallest branches, must be open to allow an unimpeded flow of blood through them. If the channel becomes narrowed at any point, not enough blood will be able to get through. If the channel is completely closed, not even a trickle of blood can go through it. This is exactly what happens in a heart attack. Such complete closure occurs, as a rule, when a blood clot forms at this narrowed down portion in a branch of the coronary artery. This blood clot, called a *thrombus,* plugs up the channel like a cork, so completely that no blood can pass through it.

Hardening of the Coronary Artery

In order to understand how this narrowing and eventual plugging up comes about, you need to know something about the structure of all arteries, including the coronary.

The artery is a hollow tube, the walls of which consist of three layers. The inside of the artery is lined with a smooth, delicate membrane, called the *intima*. The outer layer, called the *adventitia,* consists of a protective coating that gives strength to the artery. Between these two layers there is another layer called the *media,* composed of muscles that enable the artery to contract or dilate, thus regulating its caliber. The most important change that interferes with the efficiency of the coronary artery as a feed line to the heart muscle occurs in its inner layer, the intima.

Hardening of the arteries, or *arteriosclerosis,* is probably a familiar term to you. The word itself may sound somewhat forbidding, but what you may not realize is that practically every person past the age of fifty has some degree of arteriosclerosis.

There are two kinds of hardening of the arteries, and it is important to distinguish between these two forms if you wish to understand how a heart attack is brought on.

One form is the thickening and scarring of the middle layer. This is the true arteriosclerosis. The other form, called *atherosclerosis,* consists of gradual deposition of a fatty substance in the inner layer.

Because this fatty substance resembles gruel, it is called by the Greek word for gruel, *atheroma.* This fatty substance consists mainly of *cholesterol.* An answer to why cholesterol accumulates inside the coronary arteries of some persons and not of others could go a long way to explain why some persons are more prone to suffer heart attack than others.

This deposit of cholesterol is not uniform throughout the length of the coronary artery but occurs in patches, leaving the rest of it smooth and unaffected. The portion of the coronary artery that contains an atheroma becomes much narrower because the atheroma protrudes into the channel and thus reduces its caliber.

The effect of atherosclerosis of the coronary is exactly the same as deposit of lime in a water pipe. Just as less water goes through a rusted pipe, so the flow of blood through this roughened portion of the coronary is considerably diminished.

Once a deposit of cholesterol has started, it proceeds to grow even larger by accumulating more of this fatty substance, until the channel becomes so narrowed that not more than a trickle of blood can pass through it. The surface of the atheroma that protrudes into the channel is rough and irregular, and may eventually trap some blood as it flows over it. The trapped blood finally clots, and the blood clot, called the *thrombus,* so completely plugs up that portion of the coronary that not a drop of blood can get through. This plugging up of one tiny portion of the coronary artery is what causes a heart attack.

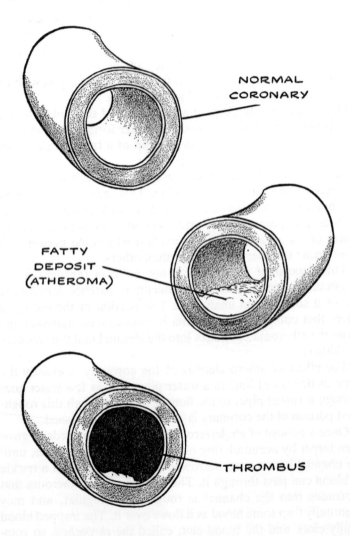

Figure 2. SECTIONS OF THE CORONARY.

Myocardial Infarct

What happens when a section of the coronary artery is plugged up?

As we have stated before, each portion of the heart muscle derives its needed blood from one of the branches of the coronary artery. If one particular branch is stoppered, that tiny section of the heart muscle literally starves until it dies out, becoming a dead tissue. This dead tissue is called a *myocardial* (heart muscle) *infarct*. Naturally, the heart containing dead tissue in its midst is unable to contract as smoothly as before. The difficulty may be so great that the heart stops altogether.

In the vast majority of cases, despite such handicap, the heart continues to function adequately, although, of course, not quite so smoothly as an intact heart. The wound itself in the heart muscle, exactly like a wound in another part of the body, heals by natural processes. Eventually it is transformed into a tiny scar, exactly as when you cut your finger.

The most critical period of this healing process is the first two weeks following a heart attack. Here is the reason why your doctor will take extra care that your heart be spared the slightest exertion during this time, so that it can obtain complete rest. After this, the healing process goes on apace. By the end of six weeks the scar is formed and strong enough to withstand more stress.

What happens to the portion of the coronary artery that had been obstructed? In time the thrombus in it may be transformed into a sort of scar tissue that will keep that portion of the artery permanently closed. Or the blood clot may gradually be absorbed, so that the channel of the artery is reopened, allowing the blood to flow through it again. This is called *recanalization*. Recanalization takes time—months and sometimes even years.

The ideal thing, of course, would be to remove the thrombus immediately after it has formed. As a matter of fact, medical science has already taken the first step toward this goal. Recently a new chemical compound, capable of dissolving a newly-formed blood clot, has been tried on a few patients, with highly

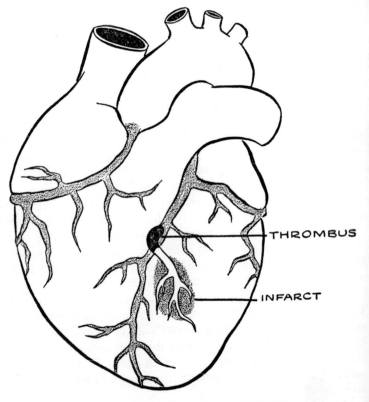

Figure 3. BLOOD CLOT IN THE CORONARY.

gratifying results in some cases. This new preparation, when it is further refined and modified, may prove to be a real miracle drug.

Fortunately, that tiny portion of the heart muscle which had been deprived of blood does not have to wait until the branch of the coronary is reopened. Very soon after a heart attack, a so-called *collateral circulation* begins to be established. Collateral circulation means that the affected portion of the heart now gets its blood from new sources.

This is accomplished in two ways. First, newly formed tiny

blood vessels sprout out from above and below the obstructed section. These newly formed blood vessels take over part of the task formerly performed by that section of the coronary artery. As a matter of fact, the now famous Beck heart operation is based on the principle of prodding the heart to form such new, tiny blood vessels.

But even more importantly, already existing tiny blood vessels connecting the larger branches begin to enlarge following a heart attack, until they are wide enough to carry as much blood to the heart muscle as it had received before the attack. Collateral circulation can be likened to a detour in traffic when the main thoroughfare is blocked off.

It takes about three weeks following a heart attack for collateral circulation to deliver enough blood so that the heart as a whole can function creditably. The new blood routes continue to enlarge, allowing more and more blood to flow through, until the damaged portion of the heart receives as much blood as it did before. That is why the majority of heart attack victims recover completely.

Coronary Insufficiency

Formation of a thrombus is not the only way by which the circulation of blood in the heart tissue is stopped. Few persons go through life without any change whatever in their coronary arteries. These fortunate few, mostly women, have exactly the same equipment in old age that they had in youth. Most of us, however, after the age of forty, begin to accumulate a few patches of cholesterol deposit in one or more parts of our coronary artery. However, these small patches do not necessarily narrow down the caliber of the artery enough to interfere with the delivery of blood to all parts of the heart.

Even though the patch does become large enough to narrow down the channel here and there, the heart can still function in a perfectly normal manner. Such is the marvelous adaptability of the heart that nature will find ways to compensate for shortcomings in one portion of it.

In one large university, out of 3,000 autopsies, the hearts of no less than 1,629 of these were found to have rather marked narrowing in one or more branches of their coronary arteries. Yet the vast majority of these persons died from some other cause. It is extremely likely that none of these persons ever knew their heart had been somewhat impaired.

Often such narrowing is quite severe. The atheromatous patches are large enough completely to stop blood flow in one or more small subdivisions of the coronary artery, yet the person can perform sometimes rather heavy work and never actually suffer a heart attack.

A person may actually sustain a very small myocardial infarct (wound) without being in the least incommoded by it and without being aware of it. Pathologists who perform large numbers of autopsies on persons who have died from some disease wholly unconnected with the heart, often find one or even more scars in the heart. Here is evidence that the person had, perhaps years ago, suffered a sudden occlusion of one branch of his coronary artery with subsequent infarction. Yet when the family is closely questioned, they state definitely that the person had never been seriously sick at any time in his life.

There is a possibility that what such a person took for an upset stomach was actually a mild heart attack. It is also possible that such mild heart attacks do not incapacitate the person. All in all, far more people than is generally realized have some degree of coronary atherosclerosis without in the least being inconvenienced by it.

However, a person who has more severe atherosclerosis of the coronary artery may be less capable of withstanding the extreme stresses and tensions of life. As long as we lead a life of moderation, without sudden strains or emergency situations, our heart, even with a severely diseased coronary, will be able to respond to ordinary demands simply because it is never called upon too suddenly to furnish more blood than the diseased coronaries are capable of delivering.

But if such a person attempts to perform some unusually heavy task, a greatly narrowed and somewhat inelastic coronary artery will not be able to deliver the extra blood which the heart at the moment is crying for. The result is that the heart muscle, or, more precisely, that portion of the heart which obtains its fuel from that particular branch of the coronary artery, becomes literally anemic. If the anemic condition continues for any length of time, while the heart attempts to work under such unfavorable circumstances, that portion dies out as surely as if the artery had been completely closed by a thrombus.

So in such cases there develops a relative insufficiency of the coronary circulation. The heart demands more blood than it can get. Even sudden death may occur. You've no doubt heard or read about elderly men who suddenly collapsed and died while shoveling snow or mowing the lawn, or after being terribly upset emotionally, or after going back to work too soon after having been laid up for a few weeks because of some other kind of indisposition. What happens in such instances is that an *already diseased* coronary becomes so overloaded that the heart stops altogether.

How emotional upset alone may cause death in persons whose coronaries had been severely damaged is illustrated by a well-known incident in the history of medicine. The famous 18th century surgeon, John Hunter, who was afflicted with severe angina pectoris, once remarked to a friend: "My life is in the hands of any scoundrel who chooses to annoy or tease me." And so it turned out, for during a medical meeting he was engaged in a heated controversy. At the height of the argument, John Hunter suddenly turned pale, collapsed, and died.

However, it must not be imagined that a sudden and acute coronary insufficiency will invariably lead to death. On the contrary, statistics show that a heart attack developed on the basis of insufficiency is far less likely to be fatal than one due to thrombosis. In several studies it was found that in contrast to the average of 10 to 15 per cent of deaths following thrombosis, the mortality rate in cases of insufficiency is less than 5 per cent.

Nevertheless, relative insufficiency is extremely important. For after recovery from either kind of heart attack, the coronary artery may remain somewhat deficient. This deficiency imposes certain limitations not only on physical activity but, perhaps even more importantly, on emotional and mental expenditure. For this reason you must learn what sort of physical or mental activity is likely to overtax the coronary in order to become adjusted to new ways of life.

3

Symptoms of Heart Attack

THERE IS ALWAYS considerable risk in describing the symptoms of any ailment. Most people reading about them invariably imagine they have just these and are naturally frightened.

This reaction is especially common in anything connected with the heart. As a matter of fact, there are a good many middle-aged men who are in such constant dread of a heart attack that they go to one doctor after another, insisting they have heart trouble. It would do such a person no good for even the best heart specialist in the world to assure him there is nothing wrong with his heart, for he is convinced the doctor either does not know what is wrong, or is hiding the facts from him. These persons, well known to all doctors, are called cardiophobiacs. Curiously, most of these cardiophobiacs do not have any heart trouble at all. The symptoms they describe are extremely vague, if not outright fantastic.

Even though you are not a cardiophobiac, you'll probably be frightened if you have a sudden stab or twinge in the region of your heart, sure you are having or are about to have a heart attack. The fact is that *pain in the chest by no means necessarily indicates a heart attack*. Physicians have described at least twenty different kinds of chest pain in no way connected with the heart. On the other hand, a true heart attack may come on in such a mild form, with vague symptoms amounting to only a momentary discomfort, that it may easily be overlooked and valuable time lost by delay in seeking medical help.

Sometimes it happens that a man has a heart attack in such a mild form that, not even suspecting it, he either continues to work or does exactly the wrong thing. One prominent heart specialist relates that once when he was called to a middle-aged man, he found his patient chinning himself from the top of the door, trying to relieve the tightness in his chest. Actually, the man was suffering from an acute heart attack.

Sometimes a person having a heart attack will thrash around in bed from side to side in an effort to find a more comfortable position, or pace the floor, or massage the front of his chest. Yet the most important thing immediately following a heart attack is *absolute rest for the heart itself,* which is an entirely different thing from rest as it is ordinarily thought of.

Although none of the usual symptoms of a heart attack necessarily means a heart attack, it is highly important for a middle-aged man to know what they are, provided he does not attempt to make a self-diagnosis and does not get scared needlessly. It is better to be on the safe side and to know when to call a doctor.

Pain

The most prominent and striking symptom of a heart attack is pain. This kind of pain is felt in the center of the chest, directly under the breast bone. It is more a feeling of an oppression and heaviness in the chest, as though a heavy weight were lying on the chest, than actual pain. It is sometimes accompanied by a burning sensation.

The intensity of the pain varies greatly from individual to individual. In some persons it is rather mild, more in the nature of a discomfort. In others, it is more severe. In a very few the pain is of a truly agonizing intensity. This depends a good deal, also, on the individual's sensitivity to pain of any kind. In some persons the threshold of pain is rather high, and they ordinarily do not experience pain of any kind. Others have a lower threshold, and feel any kind of pain to an exaggerated degree.

The main thing for you to remember is that *the intensity of the pain has nothing whatever to do with the ultimate outcome of a heart attack.* Don't think that the more severe the pain, the more severe the heart attack is. Or that if the pain is very mild it can safely be disregarded. The chances for recovery are exactly the same. A person with a truly agonizing pain has just as good a chance as the one who experiences only a mild discomfort.

Another characteristic of this kind of pain is that it is usually not continuous. At first it may be nothing more than a discomfort or a feeling of tightness. Then it eases up somewhat, only to return in a rather more severe form. In some patients, periods of pain and complete relief follow each other in regular succession, so much so that one physician described it as "labor pains of the heart." The pain lasts usually half an hour to an hour, seldom longer. After the attack is over, most patients are completely relieved of any kind of pain, although some may feel a rather vague heaviness in the chest for as long as a week.

Another highly characteristic feature of pain in heart attack is that it seldom is confined to the area of the heart itself. The pain usually "radiates," as physicians express it; that is, it spreads to the arm, most frequently to the left, less often to the right, and occasionally to both arms.

The pain may also radiate to the upper part of the abdomen. Hence it is often mistaken for acute indigestion.

Acute Indigestion

If you are middle-aged or past and suddenly develop an upset stomach, become somewhat nauseated, and have vague discomfort or even pain in the upper portion of the abdomen, you had better not try to cure it with baking soda. More often than not it is actually "indigestion," but what you think is nothing more than an upset stomach may actually be a heart attack.

For a heart attack sometimes comes on under the disguise of an upset stomach. In such case, there is usually no pain around the heart, and not even any difficulty in breathing. Unfortunately it too often happens that the patient first tries out a number of home remedies for indigestion before he calls the doctor, and consequently loses valuable time. For all heart specialists agree that *the sooner proper treatment is started, the better the chances for complete recovery.*

Statistics show that the incidence of early death from heart attack is much greater among patients whose initial symptoms had been purely abdominal—that is, at first mistaken for indigestion—than among patients whose presenting symptoms were those of a typical heart attack. This poorer showing is undoubtedly due to the fact that treatment of these patients had been unduly delayed.

But don't let these statistics frighten you into imagining that if you have a stomach upset it must surely be a heart attack. More often than not, an upset stomach may turn out to be just that. Call a doctor at once and let him decide.

Shortness of Breath

The next most frequent symptom of a heart attack is difficulty in breathing. Physicians call this difficulty *dyspnea*. The patient will be more or less short of breath, although not actually gasping.

Sometimes shortness of breath may be the greatest difficulty the patient experiences, even overshadowing pain. Or it may be the first symptom, coming on before the patient has any pain. Shortness of breath may persist even after the patient is in the hospital, although not to the same degree as at the height of the attack. By that time, of course, the physician has at his disposal effective means to relieve any difficulty in breathing.

Again, as with other symptoms of heart attack, shortness of breath from time to time does not invariably indicate heart attack. If you get out of breath on exertion, especially if you're overweight, you shouldn't at once jump to the conclusion that you're having a heart attack. If the discomfort disappears promptly after you've rested for a short time, you can be sure it was not a heart attack.

Sweating

More or less profuse sweating, together with pain and short-ness of breath, constitutes the most characteristic symptom com-bination of a typical heart attack. Along with this profuse per-spiration, a sense of weakness usually develops. Some patients feel on the verge of fainting, although very few actually do.

Shock

In some cases, these typical symptoms of heart attack are rather mild, the patient complaining of weakness, dizziness, slight nausea, or a general sick feeling. These symptoms are usually of short duration. In more severe attacks, however, the patient may go into shock and become extremely weak. Never-theless, even after profound shock, many patients recover after prompt medical care, although in such cases some degree of weakness persists for as long as a week or so.

Anxiety

Very few patients lose consciousness, either before or during an attack. A person in profound shock may be somewhat apa-thetic; nevertheless, his intellect is clear. However, even though the symptoms are rather mild, the vast majority of patients are assailed by a fear of impending death. This fear is expressed on the face of the patient. He appears anxious and fretful, his features are drawn, and he is almost always restless.

Besides the psychological basis for it, there are also some physical reasons for this fear of impending death. At the same time that the pain in the chest causes the tone of the chest mus-cles to increase, resulting in a feeling of tightness, there is usu-ally a sinking sensation in the stomach. Along with extreme weakness, a cold and clammy sensation in the extremities, and nausea, this sensation of sinking is usually interpreted by the patient as a sure sign of impending death.

But whatever the reason for it, this peculiar sense of impend-ing death is not justified. As a matter of fact, patients who have an intense fear at the time of the attack are just as likely to recover as those who take it more calmly.

What Brings on a Heart Attack

A few months ago I investigated the sudden and unexpected death of a thirty-nine-year-old man in apparently perfect health. Just a few hours before, late in the evening, he was driving home with his wife and two small children in the car. As he was approaching a bend in the road, someone in a car going in the opposite direction threw a ripe tomato at him, striking him in the face. Although he was usually a calm and even-tempered man, the incident so provoked him that he immediately turned his car around and started to chase his wanton assailant, who had sped away in the dark. In a few minutes he was forced to give up the chase and turn homeward again.

Immediately after being struck by the tomato, he complained to his wife of a sharp pain in his chest. By the time they got home he was perspiring profusely. His wife, now greatly alarmed, drove him to a hospital where, despite medical treatment, he expired in an hour or so. Autopsy showed that one portion of his coronary artery was greatly narrowed, with evidence of minute hemorrhage around the atheromatous plaque that partially obstructed that part of the coronary artery so greatly that it had brought on a heart attack with fatal consequences.

It appears that, at least in this case, it was a great emotional upset that had brought on sudden closure of an *already diseased* coronary artery.

Not so long ago a fifty-one-year-old man became involved in an altercation with a mail carrier, and the two exchanged perhaps no more than two or three blows. The fifty-one-year-old man collapsed and died almost immediately on the spot. The cause of death was established as a heart attack.

In another instance, a policeman was struck in the middle of the chest while trying to arrest a drunk. He had to struggle a good deal before he could subdue the drunk. Shortly afterward, the policeman complained of a heavy pain under the breastbone and was taken to a doctor's office. There an examination revealed that he was having a heart attack. Fortunately the policeman eventually recovered completely.

In these three cases, the conclusion seems almost inevitable that great emotional upset and unusual exertion must have brought on the heart attack.

Almost every person who ever had a heart attack will later recall in the minutest detail everything he had done on the day he was struck down. The chances are he is going to blame some unusual incident for it. He will recall, for example, that he had been working too hard at the office, was greatly upset emotionally, or irritated all day long, had too heavy a meal, had a tiff with his wife. If his heart attack awakened him from a sound sleep he is sure he must have had a frightening nightmare, for the first thing he noticed was that he broke out in a cold sweat. But if the patient himself is likely to blame some incident for the heart attack, his wife will be even more prone to do so.

Yet, if a few days after the person has been stricken the physician inquires minutely into all the circumstances, including emotional state and physical activity, more often than not he will find nothing unusual; nothing, at least, that could be directly connected with the occurrence of the heart attack. Nearly half of the persons who suffer a heart attack are asleep or resting at the time. Yet in the three cases quoted above, unusual physical exertion and severe emotional upset did precede the heart attack. The question is whether there was a causal relationship between such unusual happening and the heart attack, or whether it was simply a matter of coincidence.

Investigators collected the case histories of a number of heart attack victims in regard to the exact circumstances under which the heart attack occurred. A few years ago Dr. Arthur M. Master and Dr. Harry L. Jaffe of New York obtained the history of the activities of 1,347 heart attack victims in whom the attack was the result of closing of the coronary artery by a blood clot. In this way they knew what each patient had been doing at the time of the attack.

They tabulated their findings as follows:

TYPES OF ACTIVITY AT ONSET OF 1,347 ATTACKS
OF CORONARY OCCLUSION

	No. of attacks	%
Rest	401	29.8
Sleep	305	22.6
Ordinary mild activity	302	22.4
Walking	198	14.6
Moderate activity	117	8.7
Unusual or severe exertion	24	1.9
Total	1,347	100.0

Mild activity included dressing, conversing, taking a shower, getting out of bed, sitting in a theater, attending a meeting, doing light housework, riding in a train or bus, and waiting in a doctor's office.

Moderate activity consisted of work at a trade, such as painting, pressing, baking, or driving a car, shopping, and climbing stairs.

Unusual activity included sports, lifting or moving a load, and running.

But then, this is just about the way the average person spends a day. As Drs. Master and Jaffe stated it:

If the incidence of attacks in our series occurring during sleep, rest, mild or moderate activity, and walking, is compared with the percentage of time during the day usually spent in each category, a close correlation is found. Thus, about half the attacks began during sleep and rest and the majority of persons spend half the day in this way. Therefore, these activities may be considered coincidental. Similarly, the association of only 2% of the coronary occlusion attacks with severe exertion is also coincidental. Most persons perform some unusual effort at least several times a day, e.g., lifting a load, moving furniture, running after a bus, or parking a car in a small space. If effort were a precipitating factor in coronary occlusion, the incidence of attacks during strain should be much greater.

On the other hand, it has been definitely established that great emotional upset and unusual exertion can bring on a heart attack, *but only in persons whose coronaries are more or less damaged.* Some of the more common of such unusual exertions include pushing a stalled car, shoveling snow, lifting a heavy trunk, walking long distances uphill, and in general any kind of effort to which the person has not been accustomed. Coronary insufficiency is more likely to occur in cold weather than in warm.

If you are a middle-aged or elderly person and have become more or less sedentary, never attempt anything that requires sudden or strenuous exertion, especially if you are already tired or didn't have a good night's rest. If you become short of breath on slight exertion or on climbing stairs, it is possible, of course, that you have gained too much weight or are no longer used to any kind of physical activity. However, as time goes on if you get tired more easily until even the slightest exertion provokes shortness of breath, you had better see a doctor, for an ever-increasing intolerance for exertion may indicate a somewhat diseased coronary artery.

Whether the symptoms described here are dramatic and unmistakable, or vague and hardly suggestive at all of a heart attack, only a doctor will be able to tell whether they mean a heart attack or not. Today, physicians have devised many fine and accurate procedures that tell exactly what is happening to the patient, and even what part of the heart is affected.

Although the task is entirely up to the doctor, you should understand how he goes about making a diagnosis.

4

Diagnosis

EVERYONE is familiar with that indispensable item of every doctor's equipment, the stethoscope. This is simply a device that enables the doctor to hear more distinctly the sounds produced in the body, particularly those produced by breathing and by the working of the heart. Listening to the sounds is called medically *auscultation.*

As the heart contracts and expands rhythmically, the valves of the heart open and shut, each action producing a sound. So at each heart beat there are two audible sounds, repeated at regular intervals. If the valves are in perfect condition, as in a normal heart, the double sound produced is something like "lubb-dubb, lubb-dubb, lubb-dubb." However, if the valves either are too narrow or do not close perfectly, the sounds produced by an imperfect valve will instead be a soft hissing sound, known as a *murmur.*

A murmur means that the valves of the heart are affected, as for example in rheumatic heart disease. A murmur, however, does not necessarily mean heart disease. Very often a perfectly normal heart, for some unexplained reason, produces a murmur, yet functions in a perfectly normal manner.

The changes induced by a heart attack do not affect the valves themselves. Consequently, there will be no murmur after a heart attack. However, in most although not in all instances, the first heart sound is somewhat muffled, not quite so distinct as it had been before. But muffling of the first heart sound can occur in other conditions, so this simply offers no more than a suggestion to the examining physician. He will need a good many other signs before he can make certain that his patient has actually had a heart attack.

There is another kind of sound that may be a little more suggestive of a heart attack. This is a rubbing or scratching sound present in approximately 10 per cent of patients. The heart is enclosed in a sort of sac, like a plastic bag, known as the *pericardiac sac*. Sometimes in cases of an infarction the surface of this pericardiac sac becomes roughened so that it produces a rubbing sound. Again, however, this rubbing sound occurs in other conditions, so its presence is no more than an additional indication of a possible heart attack.

The stethoscope, contrary to the general impression that it will immediately reveal a heart attack, is actually of secondary importance in making a correct diagnosis. In contrast to the indefinite nature of the evidence furnished by the stethoscope, there are four main tests on which the physician depends to diagnose a heart attack. These are: temperature; count of white blood cells; the so-called sedimentation test; and the transaminase test.

Temperature

As we have explained in a previous chapter, the tiny section of heart muscle that is deprived of blood dies out, and this dead tissue is then carried away by the blood stream. The dead tissue is now a foreign matter, and the presence of a foreign matter of whatever nature causes the body temperature to rise. So, soon after a heart attack, usually within the first twenty-four hours, the patient will have a slight fever, seldom more than around 102° F. The temperature usually rises slightly on the second and third days and then returns to normal.

Even if the fever is slightly higher than this and lasts a little longer, it should not be cause for alarm. Patients who develop even a rather high temperature make just as good a recovery as those who have only a slight fever. Nevertheless, the length of time the fever persists offers some suggestion to the physician how large an area of the heart muscle has been destroyed. For the greater the amount of dead tissue, the longer it takes for all of it to be carried away by the blood stream. In such cases the temperature may be a little higher and may last slightly longer.

Count of White Blood Cells

You are no doubt familiar with how the doctor determines whether a patient with a sudden pain in the right side of the abdomen has appendicitis or not. When a person has appendicitis, the infecting material is carried away by the white blood cells. The white blood cells are the defending army of the body. When hostile forces invade the body the white blood cells rush to the rescue to destroy the foreign forces. In order to do this effectively their number necessarily increases. From this increased number of white blood cells the doctor knows the patient is suffering from appendicitis.

Exactly the same thing occurs when the hostile force consists of dead heart muscle tissue. The number of white blood cells increases after a heart attack. So the doctor obtains a few drops of blood and sends it to the laboratory where technicians can make an accurate count of these white blood cells. The count usually rises for the first three days, then returns to normal by the eighth day.

Sedimentation Test

Another scientific method in diagnosing heart attack also involves a laboratory blood test. This is a test to measure the rate of sedimentation of the red blood cells. The red blood cells are heavier than the whole blood. Consequently, if some blood is placed in a special kind of test tube the red blood cells begin to sink to the bottom. In practically every person who has suffered a heart attack, the red blood cells sink much more rapidly than in healthy persons. The laboratory technician, then, can measure how much time it takes for all the red blood cells to sink to the bottom of the test tube. A faster rate of sinking, or as it is called sedimentation, is another indication of a heart attack.

In contrast to fever and increase of white blood cells, this sign does not appear until after a day or so, more often after two days, but almost certainly within three days. This rather dependable timetable of the appearance of a faster sedimentation rate may permit the physician to determine the approximate time of a heart attack. For example, if at the time of his first examination of a patient the sedimentation rate is already faster than normal, the doctor is almost sure that the patient has suffered a heart attack a day or two previously, although it may have been so mild that the patient himself didn't recognize it.

This increased rate of sedimentation persists sometimes as long as thirty-six days. Persistence has no significance at all as to the severity of the attack, but the doctor can judge by it how well the patient is recovering and accordingly modify the time he must stay in bed.

Transaminase Test

There is present in all muscles of the body, and especially in the heart muscle, a chemical substance called transaminase. The amount of this substance greatly increases following a heart attack, so that a laboratory test to determine the amount of it in the blood aids the physician in making a diagnosis.

Increase of transaminase in the blood begins some six to twelve hours following a heart attack and reaches its peak in a day to a day and a half. By means of this test the physician can tell how large the infarct is. When the amount of transaminase returns to normal, the healing processes are progressing satisfactorily.

Other Tests

There are a number of other laboratory tests, even more complicated, that can tell a good deal about what is going on inside the heart. Most of these newer tests are rather expensive, and many hospitals are not yet equipped for carrying them out. If these newer methods are not used, the patient should not feel that he is not getting the most up-to-date methods to make the diagnosis absolutely sure. These newer tests are far less reliable than the four basic ones we have described, and are helpful primarily for research work. The four tests we have described are available to every patient, regardless of his purse, and can tell the physician all he needs to know to make a diagnosis.

In addition to these laboratory tests, the physician depends for diagnosis, and also as a guide to how well the patient is progressing, on the *electrocardiogram*.

The Electrocardiogram

Practically every person today is acquainted with the electrocardiogram. The instrument that takes the electrocardiogram is one of the most remarkable medical inventions, and has become today practically indispensable in accurately determining the condition of the heart.

The machine is far too complicated to be described here. However, its basic principles are not too difficult to understand. When the heart contracts it produces an electric current. However, this electric current is not a continuous one. Each part of the heart, as it contracts, successively produces its own characteristic electric impulse, differing in voltage and timing. As the impulse travels from one part of the heart to the other, the electric current thus produced follows a specific pattern. This pattern is repeated in exactly the same way with each heart beat.

Several electrodes are placed at certain points on the skin. These electrodes pick up the current produced by the contraction of the heart. The current, magnified by the machine, activates a pen which "writes" on a roll of photographic paper that moves at a uniform speed.[1] This writing—the electrocardiogram—consists of wavy lines, each section or "wave" of which

[1] Actually there are two general types of instruments: (1) direct writers which write on heat-sensitive paper that does not require developing and is activated by the heated pen; and (2) photographic instruments which record on photographic paper but which use a beam of light from an optical galvanometer or photograph the shadow of a string in a magnetic field.

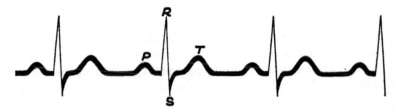

Figure 4a. ELECTROCARDIOGRAM OF A NORMAL HEART.

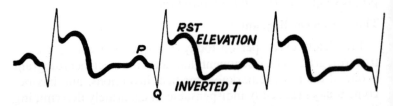

Figure 4b. ELECTROCARDIOGRAM TAKEN AFTER A HEART ATTACK.

had been produced by the contraction of different parts of the heart. After a heart attack, the pattern of the electric current—and, consequently, the electrocardiogram—changes. These changes tell the physician to what extent and even what part of the heart muscle has been affected.

To give you some idea of what an electrocardiogram looks like and how the physician interprets, or, as it is called, "reads" it, we give you here three different electrocardiograms. The first is an electrocardiogram of a normal heart; the second, taken immediately after a heart attack; and the third, about two weeks afterward.

Figure 4a represents the electrocardiogram of a normal heart. You will notice that there are elevations and dips above and below the horizontal line. Each of these recurrent waves is known by a letter, beginning with P. You will also notice that the pattern is repeated in exactly the same way, representing the rhythmic contraction of the heart.

Now let's compare this with an electrocardiogram taken shortly after a heart attack. In Figure 4b you will notice that

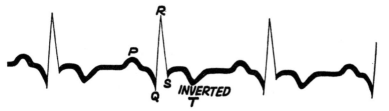

Figure 4c. ELECTROCARDIOGRAM TAKEN TWO WEEKS AFTER A HEART
ATTACK.

the pattern of these wavy lines has changed considerably. The
P wave is the same as before. However, the line between P and
T is no longer straight. There is a V-shaped dip in it called the
Q wave. Also, the line after the peak at R now does not dip
down abruptly, but there is an elevation called the RST elevation that was not present in the normal electrocardiogram. The
third point you will note is that the T wave, instead of pointing
upward, now points downward, and is called an inverted T
wave. The same changed pattern is repeated in the same way,
meaning that the heart is now contracting in a different way at
every heart beat.

These changes indicate that a heart attack has taken place.

Figure 4c is an electrocardiogram of the same person taken
about two weeks later. The heart is now mending, and so the
waves produced are beginning to return to normal, although
still not completely so. In this figure you will notice that the
RST elevation is no longer present. However, the abnormal
Q is still there, and the T wave is still inverted. These slight
changes may remain sometimes for months, even after the
heart has been completely mended.

If your physician tells you that your electrocardiogram is
still somewhat different from what it was before the heart
attack, do not be unduly frightened. There are many persons
whose electrocardiograms show an inverted T wave but who
never had a heart attack and whose heart is perfectly normal.

The physician can tell from the electrocardiogram what part

of the heart is damaged by an infarct, and he can also gather a general idea how large the infarct is. Furthermore, as the wound in the heart muscle heals, the original pattern changes, so that by taking repeated electrocardiograms he can also determine how the patient is progressing.

Although the electrocardiogram is an invaluable aid to the physician in diagnosing heart attack, and also in telling how the heart is mending, there are some popular misconceptions about it that should be dispelled at once. The average person thinks the doctor can tell everything about the condition of the heart from the electrocardiogram alone. Actually, some condition may exist that does not show on the electrocardiogram at all.

For example, a person may have a greatly narrowed coronary artery, yet his electrocardiogram may be perfectly normal. The reason for this is that there will be no changes in the pattern of the electric current until the heart muscle itself is injured.

On the other hand, a person with a perfectly normal heart may, for one reason or another, have an abnormal graph in some respect.

Furthermore, the electrocardiogram may not show any evidence of a true heart attack. Since only the outer layers of the heart muscle can be explored, damage to the deeper layers may not show at all on the electrocardiogram.

You should also bear in mind that an electrocardiogram does not give an automatic answer as to whether or not you have had a heart attack. It must be interpreted, or read, by a physician. Practically all electrocardiograms of normal persons are somewhat different, so the changes brought on by a heart attack are never exactly alike in every person.

It takes expert knowledge and a good deal of experience to read an electrocardiogram properly. Even so it is not always possible to detect damage from the electrocardiogram alone.

There is a story that is probably apocryphal, but which, nevertheless, well illustrates the popular idea that a physician supposedly can tell everything about the heart by simply glancing at an electrocardiogram.

According to this story, Dr. Paul Dudley White once visited the New York office of a famous heart specialist. As he had come unannounced, the heart specialist was not in. Dr. White wandered to the record room and, without telling who he was, asked the technician to see some of the electrocardiograms. After looking over many of them, Dr. White asked the technician what was the usual percentage of electrocardiograms the heart specialist was unable to interpret. The technician replied indignantly that this specialist could, of course, read every one of them perfectly.

"That's fine," Dr. White replied. "I have several thousand in my office that I can't read at all."

Interpretation of the electrocardiogram, naturally, is important in diagnosing and treating heart attack. Nevertheless, the physician never makes a diagnosis on the electrocardiogram alone. He will consider many other factors both in establishing a correct diagnosis and also in judging how your heart is recovering from the initial damage to it.

5

Mending of the Heart

A THREE-STAGE rocket sends a satellite orbiting around the moon. Within the satellite are delicate and complicated instruments that gather and relay back to the earth information gathered in the course of the satellite's journey in outer space.

What a marvel of scientific and engineering achievement! What a miracle of precision! The rocket itself has at least three hundred thousand parts, every single one of which must perform perfectly, exactly as calculated by the scientists who have assembled this extraordinarily complex piece of machinery. If only one smallest part fails to function properly, the whole rocket will blow up on the ground.

Yet, almost unbelievable scientific achievements though they seem, the moon rocket and its satellite are like primitive and crude toys when compared with even the tiniest of living organisms, a single cell.

Each of the cells that comprise the human body is an unbelievably complex, tiny, living matter, containing perhaps more than the three hundred thousand components of a moon rocket. And the miracle is multiplied by trillions when we consider that the human body contains trillions of cells. These trillions of cells work in unison, each performing its specific task, the sum total of which is a breathing, thinking, sentient, and living human being.

No ingenuity of man has as yet succeeded in reproducing even one of these components as they exist in the living cells, although the precise nature of many of them is known to science. And even though we may compare, in a crude way, the function of the human body with a man-made machine, in one vital respect, at least, the comparison breaks down completely. If any one of the three hundred thousand parts of the moon rocket breaks down, a mechanic must repair the broken part. In contrast to this, the human machine has its own mechanic that instantly sets to work to repair any broken down part.

Your Heart Repairs Itself

The moment you suffer a heart attack, forces present in the remotest parts of the body mobilize instantly to mend the damage sustained by the heart muscle. You are, of course, unaware of the repair work going on inside your body and, even more, that there is a definite time schedule of nature's healing processes.

The very first day after a heart attack you may feel so perfectly well and vigorous that you are likely to resent the doctor's insistence that you avoid the slightest exertion and lie quietly in bed. When he won't allow you to light a cigarette for which you are nearly dying, you think he is punishing you unnecessarily, or that he is overcautious. On the other hand, you may be terribly discouraged and despondent when you still feel weak days after a heart attack, sure that you are going to die. However, if you realize how the hidden forces of the body are mobilized to patch up, slowly but on a definite schedule, the tiny wound in the heart, you'll be more likely to follow your doctor's instructions faithfully, and so help yourself to proceed to complete recovery.

Now let's see what this time schedule is.

Time Schedule

For many years scientists have carried out detailed studies of what is happening to the heart itself and to the body as a whole when the blood supply to the heart muscle is shut off suddenly. The separate findings of all this research were integrated so successfully and so completely that it would hardly be an exaggeration to say that today we know more about the healing processes of the heart than of perhaps any other phase of man's diseases. So accurate is our knowledge about myocardial infarct that we now know exactly what is going on in the heart during the first week after a heart attack, and the subsequent changes by day and by week.

The portion of the heart muscle that has been deprived of blood begins to die out *five or six hours* after the heart attack. However, it takes about *two weeks* before every cell in the damaged area has been completely destroyed.

As soon as that tiny portion of the heart muscle begins to die out, the marvelously arranged protective forces of the body come into play. First of all, the dead tissue must be removed. This task is performed by the white blood cells. You remember that one of the ways the doctor diagnoses a heart attack is by noticing a rather sharp increase in white blood cells. The reason why there is an increase of white blood cells after a heart attack is that they are entrusted with the task of carrying away the debris.

There are a number of different kinds of white blood cells, each with a highly specialized function. At the first sign of trouble, one type of white blood cells invades the margin of the dying area and then gradually wanders wherever the cells seem to be in serious trouble. We do not know, as yet, exactly what their function is, but there are indications that this type of white blood cell delivers a yeast-like substance which softens up the dead tissue. It takes *about four days* for these white blood cells to prepare the deadened tissue for another type of white blood cells, which are the real clean-up crew.

The cells of this clean-up crew are of enormous size, as size goes in this microscopic realm. Their task is to swallow up the dead cells and carry them away into the blood stream. This clean-up crew comes on the scene on the *fifth day* after a heart attack. After *about three weeks* their task is practically over, for by that time they have carried away almost all the dead tissue. But even then, there may be some few dead cells present, so these ever-busy large white cells continue "sweeping up," until not the tiniest portion of dead tissue is left.

While this cleaning up is going on, the dead tissue is gradually replaced by new cells, forming scar tissue. This scar begins to form as early as the *third to the fifth day* after the heart attack, and continues for *two or at the most three weeks,* at the end of which time the scar will be strong enough to contract synchronously with the rest of the heart muscle. Obviously, this little wound must be carefully guarded until it is completely healed, and so no extra demand must be put upon the heart during this time.

After the wound in the heart muscle is completely healed, of course, the heart will very gradually be able to take on a little extra work, for the scar tissue strengthens slowly for *two or three months*. By that time, it has become as strong as it ever will be. This is the reason why many heart attack victims recover so completely that they are able to do anything they had done before the attack.

But the remarkable recuperative power of the body does much more than simply write off the injured area as a total loss. It provides also for the portion of the heart that has been deprived of blood by plugging up of the coronary artery. In other words, since the supply line is blocked in one direction, the body builds a new pipe line for that portion of the heart. Of all the marvelous healing powers of the human body, perhaps none is more remarkable than its ability to establish what is called collateral circulation.

Collateral Circulation

In order to understand how collateral circulation comes about, it will be profitable to review briefly how the entire heart itself is supplied with blood. The heart, like all other tissues in the body, receives nourishment from the blood stream. You are by now familiar with the coronary artery, which supplies the heart muscle with this needed nourishment. Now, as you can see in Figure 1 (page 15), there are two coronary arteries: the right and the left. Both the left and the right coronaries send out a branch that encircles the back of the heart. Each of these main branches sends out finer and finer blood vessels that honeycomb the heart muscle, so that even the smallest portions of it are supplied with blood.

In the past it was thought that these main branches and their subdivisions form a closed circuit and that no intercommunication among the subdivisions of each branch exists.

By some highly ingenious experiments, scientists succeeded in proving that there actually are connecting channels between the main branches of the coronary artery. After removing a heart in autopsy, pathologists injected a radio-opaque material into one branch of the coronary and found that the material appeared in the finer vessels of another branch. There could, then, be no question that there were fine channels connecting one branch and its subdivisions with another.

The next step was to measure the caliber of these communicating channels called collateral vessels. Scientists found that the caliber of these collateral vessels was extremely small, not much larger than that of the capillaries, those smallest subdivisions of the arteries. Still later, scientists were able to demonstrate that, unlike the capillaries, these collateral vessels do not carry blood under ordinary circumstances. These investigators then showed that in persons who had suffered a heart attack the collateral vessels immediately begin to enlarge and to carry blood. Then they grow to several times their normal size, until they are able to take over the task of the artery that had been plugged up by a thrombus. In this way, nature has provided a most ingenious arrangement to supply blood to that part of the heart muscle which was cut off from its normal supply when the person suffered a heart attack.

It would hardly be an exaggeration to say that these collateral vessels are like spare tires for a car. When your heart has a flat tire, nature rushes in spare ones to replace it.

It is not only after a heart attack that these collateral vessels open up. If some of the branches or subdivisions of the coronary artery become very much narrowed by atherosclerosis so that they are not able to carry all the blood the heart needs, these collateral vessels begin to enlarge up to several times the size of their caliber so that they supplement the capacity of the narrowed portions of the coronary.

Persons who have a highly efficient collateral circulation will never suffer a heart attack, for these spare parts are already functioning and can immediately take over if one branch does become obstructed.

You may have bad coronaries, but you may never suffer a heart attack.

Pathologists examined at autopsy the hearts of a number of older persons who had died from some other disease not connected with the heart in any way. They found that in a large proportion of these, perhaps more than half, the coronary arteries were greatly narrowed. In quite a number, one segment or even more of the coronary was actually completely closed. Yet they found no evidence of infarct in the hearts of any of these persons.

A few months ago a seventy-three-year-old man was driving along the road at a moderate speed. Suddenly, at an intersection, another car crashed through the red light and collided with the old man's car, killing him almost instantly. Autopsy revealed that he had died from severe brain injury and skull fracture.

However, the most remarkable and really astonishing thing was the condition of his coronaries. One segment, and not even a very short one, in each of the three main branches of the coronary artery was closed completely by the accumulation of fatty substances. From microscopic examination it was evident that this complete stoppage had occurred many years previously, probably on three separate occasions.

It was wonder enough to figure out how, with these complete closures in the coronary, the heart muscle could ever have got enough blood. Yet there was no old scar any place in the heart muscle. This man had been treated by a doctor over a number of years for mild diabetes, and at no time during his frequent medical examinations was any evidence found of a heart attack. His wife knew of no episode of even a mild indisposition, much less a heart attack or anything resembling it.

As his coronaries became gradually more and more narrowed, a highly efficient collateral circulation was developed over the years, and his heart received enough blood at all times. Each time one segment of the coronary became completely closed, his collateral circulation was already so well established that the blood was shunted into these spare channels. Consequently the man never suffered a heart attack.

But the real surprise was yet to come. The autopsy also showed that in one small branch of his coronary artery there was a fresh blood clot that had been there perhaps a day or two.

On this fatal drive he had just come from his doctor's office for a checkup for his diabetic condition. He had not complained of any chest pain at that time. His wife later stated that for the past two or three days he had been in his usual health. If anything, the very fact that he was able to drive his car proves that he was in no way affected by the thrombus. That he did not suffer a heart attack at this time either, despite the presence of a blood clot, again shows the effectiveness of his collateral circulation.

This case, of course, is extraordinary. Nevertheless, the fact is that only a small percentage of all persons who have greatly narrowed coronaries ever suffer a heart attack. Obviously, the vast majority of persons with diseased coronary arteries develop a highly efficient collateral circulation. Consequently, if a person suffers a heart attack he did not have an efficient collateral circulation, at least in that portion of the heart. If he did not have it before, however, the heart attack itself induces development of collateral circulation at that particular point. Immediately after a heart attack, these previously existing but unused collateral vessels begin to enlarge and to open for the flow of blood through them. In two or three weeks they will become large enough to carry a sufficient amount of blood to the heart muscle for it to function normally again.

Scientists have shown that, if the area of the heart muscle which has been deprived of blood is very small, absolute rest until efficient collateral circulation develops may prevent the affected portion of the heart muscle from dying out altogether. That is to say, in such cases no infarct will appear. Naturally, the affected portion of the heart muscle will receive a reduced amount of blood, but even this reduced amount will be sufficient to allow this tiny portion of the heart muscle to stay alive until it receives enough blood by means of collateral circulation.

Besides utilizing these already existing channels to establish collateral circulation, nature has another and even more remarkable way of restoring integrity to a damaged heart. This is the extraordinary ability of the heart muscle to sprout entirely new, even though extremely small, blood vessels as a means of helping out the damaged one.

These new blood vessels begin to form as early as the fourth day after a heart attack, and each day thereafter their number multiplies. By the end of twelve days they are sturdy and capable of functioning effectively. After three weeks, they and the collateral vessels, are almost as effective as the closed up portion of the coronary had been. But this is not all. These newly-formed blood vessels continue to sprout additional new branches for as long as one year after a heart attack.

Most people think that the heart of a person who has had a heart attack will become weaker and weaker as time goes on. Actually, the opposite is true. Because of this sprouting of additional blood vessels and the consequent additional supply of blood to the heart muscle, the heart of such a person becomes stronger, instead of weaker, with time.

The practical significance of nature's timetable in mending a damaged heart is this: During the first two or three weeks after a heart attack, while collateral circulation is being established and before the scar has had time to become strong and firm, it is absolutely necessary that the heart remain at complete rest and that no extra burden be imposed on it. The oxygen carried by the blood during this time will be just enough to maintain the work of the heart for the basic functions of the body. Any added burden on the heart, obviously, will use up more oxygen, so that the supply may become insufficient for vital life processes.

6

Treatment

THE FIRST THING the average person does if someone in the family becomes suddenly ill is to rush him to the hospital. The family, naturally frightened, call frantically for an ambulance. If it does not arrive at once, they call again and again—it's a matter of life or death. If someone happens to think about it, he may call the doctor, but likely as not the doctor doesn't learn about the trouble until the patient has already arrived at the hospital.

The ambulance attendants, trained for emergency, will carefully place the victim on a stretcher and carry him to the ambulance with as little jarring as possible. But once in the ambulance, the helpless patient is rushed at breakneck speed through the traffic, siren screeching, racing to beat death by a nose.

Actually, in the great majority of cases, this frantic speed is not only completely unnecessary but is often the worst possible thing for the patient himself. Recently Drs. George J. Curry and Sydney N. Lyttle of Flint, Michigan, analyzed 2,500 consecutive ambulance runs that had been made to the hospital. They found that in the great majority of cases (98.2 per cent) rush had been absolutely unjustified. In the other 1.8 per cent, quick handling was necessary but, even in these cases, first aid at the scene would have been much better than rushing the patient to the hospital.

So senseless and completely unfounded is this general idea of rush that Dr. Basil C. MacLean, New York City Commissioner of Hospitals, has half-jocularly remarked: "The average patient would get there soon enough by parcel post."

The needlessness of rush applies especially to the victim of a heart attack. What an injured heart needs above all is rest, absolute rest. The heart must be relieved of any work and expenditure of energy. The excitement and the confusion of the family, and the inevitable commotion attending the patient's removal from his home, are the very conditions likely to increase the work of an ailing heart. Added to this, the mental anguish the heart attack victim must suffer when he is led to believe that he is regarded as near death will inevitably increase the load on the heart.

Never rush a heart attack victim to the hospital. Instead, call your doctor. He will tell you exactly what to do. Naturally, it would be asking the impossible for a wife not to be greatly upset when she sees her husband struck down in seemingly perfect health. Nevertheless, coolness, calmness, and efficient help at the moment of need will be a tremendous help.

The victim should be put to bed at once, the pillow under his head raised, his necktie opened, and he should be made generally as comfortable as possible. Don't ever give him any kind of medicine, although about an ounce of whiskey may ease his pain a bit. When the doctor arrives he will give the patient an injection to ease his pain.

It isn't always necessary to take the patient to the hospital. Very often, depending on what the doctor prefers in the individual case, the patient can be very effectively treated at home.

If the doctor does decide the case can be more safely and efficiently treated in a hospital, he will never allow the patient to be removed from the home until he has quieted down somewhat and has attained a more restful state.

Hospital care, of course, has many advantages. The doctor can follow your progress much more closely in the hospital.

Nurses and internes, as well as all hospital facilities, are immediately available for any emergency. The hospital regimen will enforce compliance with the doctor's instructions, which the patient in his own home might be tempted to disregard.

If the patient is to remain at home, he must follow strictly and accurately the same regimen he would have to observe in the hospital. The patient, as well as the family, must fully understand what the doctor is trying to achieve and the reason behind each step, so that he will cooperate willingly and not try to cheat or skip certain instructions.

On the other hand, even if the patient is being treated in a hospital, the doctor or the nurse cannot watch him every minute, and for at least part of each twenty-four hours he will be on his own. The hospital patient, also, should become fully acquainted with details of the treatment and reasons for specific instructions, so that he will follow them willingly and not think the doctor is being unnecessarily strict.

Pain Relief

The first thing the physician will do is to give an injection to relieve the victim's pain. This relief from pain serves a double purpose. First, it calms the patient and reduces restlessness, unnecessary fretting, and frequent turning in the bed, all of which are harmful for the injured heart. In the second place, the most frequently used pain killer, morphine, also has the effect of enhancing the patient's sense of well-being and thus removes some of the overwhelming fear of impending death so apt to follow a heart attack. The physician usually gives a quarter grain of morphine, but if the pain is more intense he may double the dose. However, since morphine has a tendency to depress respiration, for patients who have difficulty in breathing he may prefer to use other narcotic drugs, such as demerol. Doctors sometimes find it necessary to give narcotic medication intravenously, so that the effect will appear immediately instead of after the ten to 20 minutes required for a subcutaneous injection to take effect. Later, when the patient is in the hospital and still has pain, the doctor may give narcotics from time to time in very small doses, but this is very seldom necessary.

Oxygen

Especially on the first few days after a heart attack, the doctor may prescribe air greatly enriched in oxygen content. Most people think that when a person is placed in an oxygen tent he is actually breathing in pure oxygen. Although pure oxygen is sometimes used for short periods of time, it cannot be used for any considerable length of time because it causes irritation of the lungs. What is actually meant by oxygen treatment is that the air the patient inhales contains up to 70 per cent of oxygen, the upper limit that can be used safely for a prolonged time. As a matter of fact, most patients do not need even that much. A concentration of 45 to 50 per cent is usually sufficient.

The changes effected by oxygen are often dramatic. Many heart attack victims become blue in the face or, as it is termed medically, cyanotic. With oxygen, the patient regains a healthy color often in a very short time. The breathing of some persons is rather labored after heart attack, a condition called medically dyspnea. Oxygen is highly effective in relieving dyspnea.

Another remarkable effect of oxygen is that it has a tendency to slow the heart down to normal. Blood pressure, which is likely to fall to a low level shortly after a heart attack, rises to a safer level and soon becomes normal under its influence.

Obviously, the infarct itself, that small area in the heart muscle that has been completely deprived of blood, cannot possibly derive any benefit from an increased amount of oxygen. However, the blood flow to the area of the heart muscle surrounding the infarct has been greatly diminished after the heart attack, and so it is here that the increased oxygen content of the blood compensates for the decreased flow. This added oxygen can help prevent the wound in the heart muscle from spreading.

Administering Oxygen

The most satisfactory way to give oxygen is by means of an oxygen tent, although it can also be given either by mask or nasal catheter. One advantage of the tent is that both temperature and humidity can be regulated, especially important in uncomfortably hot weather. Temperature is usually maintained at a constant level of 60° F. to 68° F., with low humidity. Nowadays, small plastic face tents are available for home use.

Sometimes, however, an oxygen tent is not feasible, in which case other methods of giving oxygen are available, and in some cases preferable. One method is using a mask. Oxygen also can be given through a nasal catheter connected to the tank. These latter two methods are most often used if hospitalization is not needed or is, for some reason, unavailable. Even in the hospital the attending physician may prefer to use either a mask or nasal catheter instead of a tent, at least for short periods of time, since by these methods the concentration of oxygen can be considerably increased. However, most persons poorly tolerate a nasal catheter and may become so irritated by it that it will have to be dispensed with altogether.

At any rate, if for some reason or other neither hospitalization nor oxygen in any form is available, the patient and his family should not think that he is not getting the best medical treatment. For helpful as oxygen treatment is, it is not absolutely indispensable, and in many cases it is not needed at all. As it is, a large scale study has indicated that only about 60 per cent of all heart attack patients ever need oxygen in any form.

How long the patient will need oxygen depends on his condition. As a rule, four or five days will be sufficient, and very seldom is it needed the second week. But even if your doctor prescribes oxygen after this period, you should not think that your condition is particularly severe. There may be some minor complication for which you still need oxygen, even though the wound in your heart is healing satisfactorily.

When the doctor judges that you no longer need oxygen he will not stop it abruptly. So that you will become accustomed to breathing room air again he will order gradual reduction of oxygen concentration until it attains the level of oxygen in the air, which is approximately 20 per cent.

Useful and definitely helpful as oxygen is in the treatment of heart attack, one widespread popular misconception about its use in general should at once be dispelled. When the average person learns that a patient has been placed under an oxygen tent, for whatever reason, he immediately concludes that oxygen is being used as a last resort and that the patient must be on the danger list. Actually, it means nothing of the sort. Oxygen is given simply to make the patient more comfortable or to relieve some attending symptom of his ailment. It is also used for many other conditions. For example, an asthmatic patient may be placed temporarily under an oxygen tent to make his breathing easier, yet he certainly is in no danger of his life.

Nevertheless, perhaps because oxygen therapy is comparatively new, or because the apparatus is imposing and somewhat mysterious, or even more because the patient is now in a completely artificial atmosphere, the average person entertains false notions about it. But what is worse, the patient himself has the same idea and inevitably thinks his days are numbered. So especially for the heart attack victim, who is more likely to become obsessed with fear of death than a patient with any other kind of ailment, it is highly important for him to know that just because he has been placed under an oxygen tent he is not necessarily dangerously ill.

Rest

Rest still remains the most efficient means the physician employs to tide the patient over the most critical period of his ailment. But rest for recovering from a heart attack is by no means the same as it is usually understood. As a matter of fact, under certain circumstances bed rest may actually increase the work of the heart.

Armchair Treatment

Since it would obviously be impossible to put the heart in a splint, as in the case of a broken bone, the next best thing is to reduce the load on the heart to the absolute minimum. However, studies made some dozen years ago showed that lying flat in bed, instead of decreasing the work of the heart, under certain circumstances may actually increase it. Some physicians began to question whether lying flat in bed for a prolonged length of time is what the patient actually needs.

The real pioneer of this truly radical change in the treatment of heart attack was Dr. Samuel A. Levine of Boston. Dr. Levine has shown that when the person lies motionless on his back the amount of blood that is returned to the heart with each beat is considerably greater than when he is in an upright position. If he is on his feet, sheer force of gravity tends to increase the amount of blood in the lower extremities. Consequently, the amount of blood that goes back to the heart from the lungs will be proportionately less. However, in the reclining position this proportion is reversed, with the result that the heart now receives more blood at each heart beat and so must work that much harder. This, of course, is exactly the opposite of what the patient actually needs.

Dr. Levine introduced what he called the Armchair Treatment. He had a few heart patients who, treated in the customary way of having the patient lie flat on his back, were rapidly getting worse. He decided to place these patients cautiously in an armchair. The improvement was immediate and nothing short of dramatic.

Encouraged by this gratifying experience of rapid improvement in these seriously ill patients, Dr. Levine and his coworkers applied the same treatment to 81 other patients, some of whom were near death. In practically every case the results were extraordinarily good. Far from their condition being aggravated, all the patients in a remarkably short time were relieved from difficulty in breathing; in some the effects were astonishing.

One sixty-year-old man, for example, acutely ill after suffering a heart attack, had become semi-conscious and was rapidly declining. Some forty hours after his heart attack he was carefully taken out of bed and placed in an armchair. His condition began to improve almost immediately. On the twenty-first day after the attack he was able to walk about his hospital room. He was dismissed on the twenty-ninth day, well on the way to complete recovery.

Not the least of the excellent results noted by these doctors was the almost miraculous effect on the patient's morale. Imagine a vigorous and active middle-aged man suddenly struck down with a heart attack. He is immediately put to bed and forbidden even the slightest movement, and is told that he must remain flat on his back for a long time. No wonder he thinks he is close to death. He feels completely helpless and has no way of judging whether he is getting better or worse. He unavoidably becomes overanxious. Anxiety, as actual measurements have shown, markedly increases the work of the heart.

However, if the patient is allowed to sit up in an armchair for gradually increasing periods he feels that he is making some progress. And what is even more important for his morale, he is sure that he is now doing something positive toward his own recovery.

Later detailed studies completely confirmed the beneficial effects of the Armchair Treatment. In 1954, Dr. W. S. Coe made an extended study of the working of the heart in six patients after a heart attack. He found that when the patient was sitting up in a chair, the volume of blood returned to the heart at each beat was considerably less than when he was lying flat on his back. On the average the difference amounts, almost unbelievably, to considerably more than a pint per minute. Therefore, since the heart received more blood in the reclining position it had to pump more blood out into the body, and so had to work that much harder. Dr. Coe calculated that the work of the heart in the sitting position was reduced no less than 23 per cent.

Following the pioneer work of Dr. Levine and his co-workers, and further convincing examples, the method of Armchair Treatment is now universally accepted by all doctors. Nevertheless, even though this new method is an extremely important step forward, you must not imagine that Armchair Treatment must be used in every case. Some patients are too gravely ill to permit any movement, while others may not need it at all. It depends altogether on the need of the individual and on his present condition. Dr. Milton Plotz, Professor of Medicine at State University of New York, estimates that about half of the patients need Armchair Treatment.

On the average, after the initial absolute bed rest, the patient is allowed to get into an armchair twenty-four to forty-eight hours after a heart attack. This does not mean that he will get there under his own power—that would put too much strain on his heart. Instead, he is helped by an attendant on each side to sit up at the edge of the bed with his legs dangling. Then the attendants place him gently in an armchair next to the bed. He is allowed to sit there for some time, until he feels just the slightest fatigue, never long enough to get tired. Care is taken that the back of the knees and calves do not press against the chair, lest the circulation in the legs be impeded. This seemingly minor point is actually an extremely important one throughout the entire period of Armchair Treatment and even later, when the patient is allowed to sit up in a chair, for it is necessary that the circulation be maintained freely at all times.

The next day, and each day thereafter, the patient will undoubtedly be able to sit in the armchair a little longer, until the day finally comes when he will be allowed to take a few steps about the room. A day or so after being allowed to sit in the armchair, the patient will be able to feed himself and to comb his hair, but not to shave.

Later, a modification of the original Armchair Treatment was introduced by Dr. J. R. Beckwith and his associates. In cases where Armchair Treatment is deemed advisable, for the first three days the patient stays in the armchair for thirty minutes, three times a day. For the next three days he is encouraged to stay there for a full hour, three times a day. For the next six days, each period is increased to an hour and a half. After this, the patient may sit in the armchair as often and for as long as he wishes. The reports on this modification are highly enthusiastic, with not a single mishap or drawback.

However, when the patient who is treated by the armchair method gets to the point where he is allowed to sit in the armchair for long periods of time, he must be cautioned about one thing. Many patients think that if they are allowed to sit in an armchair they should also be able to walk around a bit. Armchair Treatment does not mean license to take even a few steps. The patient must understand that the true basis of the Armchair Treatment is to afford maximum rest for the heart. Being in an armchair is for him exactly the same thing as being in bed. If the patient needlessly exerts his heart by taking even a few steps, all that his heart has gained will be dissipated by the completely unnecessary extra burden that walking involves.

Surgical beds can serve the same purpose as the armchair. These beds permit raising of the head and lowering of the legs, and they are available not only in hospitals but for private rental as well. Even an ordinary bed can serve the same purpose. The head end of the bed can be raised by the use of a nine-inch wooden block placed under the head post. A board or a box at the foot of the bed is useful in preventing the patient from sliding forward.

Care of the Bowels

Straining at stool puts a dangerous burden on the work of the heart and should be strictly guarded against. For the first two or three days after a heart attack the patient usually does not have any bowel movement, but this is unimportant. After a few days a small enema may be given every other day, or the physician may prescribe a very mild laxative, perhaps a teaspoonful of milk of magnesia after each meal, if necessary.

Bathing

In the hospital, tub bath is not allowed for the first five weeks. Instead, the nurse will give you a bed bath for the first three weeks, after which you will be able to bathe yourself in bed. If you are released from the hospital before this time, the practice of bed-bathing should be continued at home. Your wife, of course, can learn how to do this without involving unnecessary movement on your part.

Diet

As long as you're in the hospital, the attending physician will prescribe a suitable diet. When you are ready to be released he will give you strict instructions about what regimen to follow, and will probably use a salt-free diet.

Contrary to general impression, coffee is allowed in moderation. Also, whiskey or beer is often beneficial because of its soothing effect, especially for elderly patients who complain of weakness or are unduly depressed.

How Long You'll Have to Stay in Bed

Scientists have proved by laboratory experiments on animals that in order for a firm and resistant scar to be formed, the heart must be spared as much extra work as possible. These scientists produced infarcts in the hearts of dogs by artificial means. Then they allowed one group of dogs to rest following the infarct, while another group was exercised. In the group that had been allowed to rest, investigators found that the resulting scar was strong, small, and firm. But in those dogs that had been exercised shortly after the formation of the infarct, the scar was so thin and weak that the heart muscle in that portion was actually bulging.

Consequently, every victim of a heart attack, whether it had been mild or more severe, should rest for at least six weeks, the length of time it takes for the wound to heal completely and a firm scar to be formed.

This six weeks of bed rest is divided into two periods. During the first three weeks, while collateral circulation is being established, the patient is not allowed to walk at all. But even during these first three weeks, rest does not mean that the person should be absolutely motionless during all this time. On the contrary, complete restriction of all movements in bed beyond the first day or two following a heart attack will actually be harmful. During complete and motionless rest the circulation slows down considerably, favoring the formation of blood clots in the veins of the lower extremities, especially in older persons.

Consequently, during the first three weeks, the patient is allowed to move more or less freely in bed and to feed himself. In order to improve the circulation in the legs, the patient should bend his knees and flex his feet for a few minutes several times a day, but on a definite schedule in order to avoid becoming too tired. Elastic bandage on the legs will help greatly to improve circulation. To prevent development of painful shoulders the patient should rotate his arms a few times three or four times a day. If he is being treated at home his wife should be instructed to massage his arms and legs gently.

At the beginning of the fourth week the patient will be allowed to get out of bed and take a few steps to a comfortable chair near the bed. Each day, then, he will walk a little more, and will be allowed to stay out of bed and sit in a chair for gradually and cautiously increased periods of time. Nevertheless, he will still have to use the bedside commode.

Six weeks after the heart attack the patient is allowed to leave his room.

This six-weeks' schedule applies to the average patient. The physician will modify these general rules according to individual needs. If he determines that the attack had been an extremely slight one he may let the patient get up as early as the second or third day. On the other hand, he may decide from the various laboratory tests that the patient needs to stay in bed a little longer. In any case, your doctor will judge your case according to your own needs. If he insists that you stay in the hospital longer than you expected, don't be discouraged. It does not necessarily mean that your case is a particularly severe one.

What you need above all is to follow your doctor's instructions faithfully and unquestioningly. And don't try to cheat. As Dr. Robert Wartenberg wrote in that letter to his fellow-physician who had suffered a heart attack:

> In the acute stage, put yourself completely at the mercy of your doctor. Tell him you are not an M.D., but a plain patient. Never press him, urge him, or try to influence him. Obey him and that's all.

At the beginning of the seventh week, the heart attack victim is well on his way to recovery, and he can be regarded as a convalescent. He is then ready to work gradually toward establishing a normal schedule.

Rest for the Mind

It would be almost impossible for the person who is struck down with a heart attack in the midst of vigorous health not to be frightened and assailed by great anxiety. The physician who is called in can do a great deal to allay his anxiety and ease his mind. Of course, this is no time to explain to him what a heart attack implies. A little later, however, fully knowing that the chances of recovery are excellent, the physician can truthfully give reassurance without in the least minimizing the serious implications of a heart attack.

Fortunately, the human mind, as well as the body, is by nature very resilient. As soon as the pain eases and strength begins to return, most patients gradually overcome their preoccupation with death. Human nature being what it is, the patient will begin to worry about something else. He will become anxious about the future—the financial burden his sudden illness involves, his ability to return to work, and his earning capacity. It is exactly at this time that the patient is likely to experience his greatest mental anxiety. This, of course, can only add to the burden of an injured heart. The physician will be able to tell him, without in the least exaggerating, that the vast majority of persons who have completely recovered from a heart attack are able to return to their former occupations.

As the patient becomes less and less preoccupied with his own condition, he will become more interested in other things. This change of attitude is all to the good, for it means that he is beginning to regain his zest for life. At the same time he may become bored and restless by being confined to his room. It is exactly here that the average patient needs a word of warning.

The attending physician will, of course, forbid visitors at least for several days, depending on the circumstances. Later, however, as the patient's physical and mental condition improve, both he and his family are likely to encourage friends and business associates to visit him. Some contact with other people is desirable and even necessary in helping maintain a favorable mental attitude, but too much stimulation provided by visitors can be exhausting for the patient.

On the other hand, if friends and relatives are over-solicitous and show too much concern, the patient may come to consider himself more ill than he actually is.

So it is vitally important, if the person is treated at home, that well-meaning friends not be allowed to visit him too often or stay too long. Above all, business associates should never bring him reports from the office or expect him to transact part of his business at home.

7

The Anticoagulants

WHILE the heart itself is the chief healer of any damage it has suffered, the physician will not leave everything to nature or to chance. There are a great number of drugs that he can use to help restore any kind of derangement, whether slight or somewhat more serious, in the rhythmical contraction of the heart under altered conditions.

The doctor will watch closely the progress of your recovery and use whatever medication is needed to forestall any complications. You can rest assured that the physician has at his disposal a number of preparations that admirably accomplish this purpose according to individual needs. None of these drugs acts directly on the injured portion of the heart muscle. However, they are extremely important as an aid in maintaining the integrity of the working of the heart.

In the past few years, however, an entirely different kind of drug, which acts directly on the process responsible for a heart attack, was introduced. These drugs practically revolutionized the treatment of heart attack. Because they are capable of interfering with the clotting (coagulation) of the blood, they are called *anticoagulants.*

You will recall that the majority, but not all, of heart attacks are brought on by the formation of a blood clot in one branch of the coronary artery. Once a blood clot has formed, there is always a possibility that the blood reaching the thrombus will also become clotted, thus enlarging the original thrombus. Naturally, the larger the obstructed portion of the coronary artery the larger will be the resulting damage to the heart muscle.

But this is not the only possibility. As a rule one or more portions in other branches of the coronary artery are greatly narrowed down, but not yet completely obstructed. While the person is recovering from the first heart attack he may suffer a second heart attack from a newly formed blood clot in that other narrowed portion of the coronary.

Recent research work has shown that the blood of most persons who have severe atherosclerosis of the coronary artery has a tendency to clot more easily and more readily than the blood of healthy individuals. Ever since heart attack was first fully recognized, only a little more than forty years ago, and especially since the true nature of the disease became more accurately known, physicians realized that a drug that could prevent clotting of the blood would be a tremendous step in preventing the occurrence of either of these possibilities. But at that time medical science knew of no chemical that could perform this near miracle. Then in the early 1920's some startling discoveries were made that eventually led to the development of such near-miracle drugs.

Heparin

Ability of the blood to clot is a defense mechanism of the body to prevent the loss of too much blood. When you cut your finger, in a few minutes the blood at the point of the cut will solidify (coagulate) and plug up the tiny hole in the blood vessel so you won't lose more blood.

Clotting is the result of a rather complicated chemical reaction of the blood itself. All substances necessary for clotting are present in the blood as it circulates inside the blood vessels. When clotting is called for, these various substances set up a chain reaction, each substance being necessary for the next step, until a firm plug is formed, ordinarily a matter of a few minutes. Heparin prevents clotting of the blood by destroying one link in the chain.

Dicumarol

Here is a story of a "miracle in a haystack," in a very literal sense. It began on a bitterly cold Saturday afternoon in February, 1933, in the chemical laboratory of Dr. Karl Paul Link of the Agricultural Department of the University of Wisconsin. While a blizzard was howling and the temperature was near zero, Ed Carlson, a farmer from Deer Park, Wisconsin, some 190 miles from Madison, arrived at the laboratory. He had with him a dead heifer, a milk can of the dead animal's blood that would not clot, and about one hundred pounds of sweet clover that he used in feeding his cattle. He wanted to know what his heifer had died from.

In the early 1920's a new disease had appeared among the cattle on the prairies of North Dakota and Alberta, Canada. Animals feeding on sweet clover became progressively weaker and died in a month or two from uncontrollable internal bleeding. Two veterinarians, after extensive research, found that the blood of the dead animals lacked one of the links in the chemical chain needed for its clotting. By further search they found that only improperly cured hay, made from the common variety of sweet clover, destroyed this link in the animal's blood. From this fact they named the malady "sweet clover disease." But what was in the spoiled hay that had this effect on the blood, they did not know. All they could tell the farmers was that they must stop using spoiled clover for feed.

Late in December of 1932 Mr. Carlson lost two young heifers. On the first day of the new year, one of his favorite old cows began to bleed internally and died shortly afterward. Finally, the Friday before Mr. Carlson came to Dr. Link's laboratory, two young cows died and the bull was bleeding from the nose.

The local veterinarian told him that his cattle had died from sweet clover disease. But Mr. Carlson doubted the diagnosis. He had been feeding his cattle sweet clover for years and until then had never had any trouble. The next day he took one of the dead heifers, with a sample of its blood and the sweet clover he had been using, to the Agriculture Department of the University. The office of the State Veterinarian was closed, and by pure chance he came to the chemical laboratory of Dr. Link.

After hearing his story, Dr. Link agreed with the diagnosis of the veterinarian. But he had to tell Mr. Carlson that the only advice he could give was to stop feeding his cattle with that hay. As for the sick cattle, he might save some of these by giving them blood transfusions. Some day, perhaps in five or ten years, science might give better advice, but not now. So about four o'clock in the afternoon, the dejected Mr. Carlson took off in the still-raging blizzard for his home.

At the interview with the farmer, Dr. Link's senior student, Eugen Wilhelm Schoeffel, who had come to the United States seven years previously with a diploma in Agricultural Chemistry, had been present. Schoeffel was a highly competent chemist, cultured, fond of quoting from German poets, Shakespeare, and the Bible, intensely interested in the human side of his science. He still spoke English with a gutteral German accent.

But let Dr. Link tell the rest of the story:

"After farmer Carlson left, Schoeffel stormed back and forth in the laboratory shouting,

" 'Vat da Hell, a farmer shtruggles nearly two hundred miles in dis Sau-wetter, driven by a shpectre and den has to go home vit promises dat might come true in five, ten, fifteen years, maybe never. Who knows? Get some good hay—transfuse. Ach! Gott, how can you do dat ven you haf no money?' he snarled.

"He dipped his hands into the milk can repeatedly and while rubbing them muttered, 'Dere's no clot in dat blook! *Blut, Blut, verfluchtes Blut*. Die Menschen dauern mich in ihren Jammertagen.' (*Faust,* Prologue, line 297)

"Then, 'Vat vill he find ven he gets home? Sicker cows. And ven he and his good voman go to church tomorrow and pray and pray and pray, vat vill dey haf on Monday? MORE DEAD COWS! He has no udder hay to feed—he can't buy any. And if he loses de bull he loses his seed. Mein Gott! Mein Gott! Vy didn't ve anti-shi-pate dis? Ya, ve should haf anti-shi-pated dis.'

"We took the blood and hay and played about with them until about 7:00 P.M., when I headed for home. As I left the laboratory, Schoeffel grabbed me by the shoulders, looked me squarely in the face and said, 'Before you go let me tell you something. Der is a deshtiny dat shapes our ends, it shapes our ends I tell you! I vill clean up and gif you a document on Monday morning.' "

On that Monday, Dr. Link with his associates, including Schoeffel, began an intense search to find the mysterious substance in the spoiled hay. They gave a name to this unknown substance—the hemorrhagic agent, or the H.A. for short.

The researchers worked arduously to find the mysterious H.A. They collected balefuls of spoiled sweet clover, subjected it to all imaginable chemical tests, made extracts of it, separated, isolated, as a matter of fact did everything the chemist does to track down an unknown substance. They found many substances which they believed to be the one they were seeking, but none of them proved to be the H.A.

Finally, in the early dawn of June 28, 1939, six years and four months after that fateful afternoon, after working all night one of the researchers, Campbell, saw a tiny crystal on the microscopic slide he had prepared from the spoiled hay. It was extremely small, and it took him another two hours before he was able to collect a few more crystals. He was sure now that he had at last found the needle in the haystack. But he did not want to tell anybody before he made sure that those tiny crystals were actually the elusive H.A.

Early the next morning when Dr. Link reached the laboratory, he found Campbell asleep on the laboratory couch, the door of the room guarded by Chet Boyles, a soldier of fortune who assisted Campbell in his work. Boyles was taking a nip, as Dr. Link described it, "from the contents of a bottle whose bottom layer consisted of carpet tacks, the upper layer of 95 per cent ethanol." In non-chemical language, ethanol is simply pure alcohol. Boyles greeted Dr. Link with the words: "I'm celebrating, Doc. Campbell has hit the jackpot."

Campbell avoided Dr. Link for two days, when chemical assay showed definitely that the crystal was actually the H.A. Dr. Link, on confirming Campbell's finding, immediately sent a telegram to Schoeffel, who by that time was in charge of the chemical laboratory of the American Medical Association in Chicago. He sent back a telegram of 200 words in which he expressed his complete confidence in Nature, Fate, and the team of Dr. Link.

It was ten months later, on April Fool's Day, 1940, that a chemist in Dr. Link's laboratory announced that he had succeeded in analyzing the exact chemical structure of the substance, which turned out to be a derivative of a chemical substance present in unspoiled sweet clover, called *coumarin*, which gives sweet clover its aroma. This new chemical received the name of *dicoumarin*, and it is known today as *dicumarol*. After this, it was not long until chemists were able to make it in large quantities, and therefore inexpensively, from coal tar.

This solved the problem of Mr. Carlson and other farmers, eliminating this hazard in animal husbandry. But far more importantly, the extraordinary discovery proved to be an unexpected boon to human beings.

As soon as the discovery became known, physicians recognized immediately that the new chemical could be a valuable drug in treating human beings. The development of this safe and inexpensive drug capable of decreasing the tendency of the blood to clot was hailed enthusiastically by the medical profession. Such a drug was sorely needed, especially in preventing blood clot formation in surgical cases. Many surgeons began to use dicumarol after operation and were highly gratified to find that this formerly dreaded complication was reduced practically to the vanishing point.

At the same time, a few heart specialists gave dicumarol to patients who had suffered a heart attack, in order to forestall the occurrence of a second heart attack. Highly encouraging reports began to appear in medical literature, but the cases were still very few, and so a valid comparison of the outcome in heart patients who received dicumarol and those who did not could not be made.

You are no doubt familiar by this time with the term "control group." This means that physicians give a new drug to a number of patients, called the treated group, and withhold it from approximately the same number of patients suffering from the same disease, known as the control group. By comparing the outcome of the disease in these two groups, they are able to determine whether or not the drug is really effective. And this is what the investigators did with respect to dicumarol.

In the spring of 1946, Dr. Irving S. Wright of New York, the pioneer in the use of dicumarol in heart attack, set up a carefully planned and strictly controlled study with the cooperation of sixteen hospitals all over the country. All the patients admitted to these participating hospitals on odd days received the usual treatment but were also given dicumarol. This was the treated group. Patients admitted on even days received exactly the same treatment but did not receive dicumarol. The latter constituted the control group.

At the end of two years, there were 589 patients in the treated group and 442 in the control group, making it possible to compare a sufficiently large number of patients to allow a valid conclusion. At the end of the study the results were published. The main conclusions were these:

1. Use of dicumarol reduced the mortality rate by at least one-third.
2. The incidence of further clotting of the original thrombus and the appearance of new clots in other parts of

the coronary or some other blood vessel was reduced by more than two-thirds.

Thus, the beneficial effect of anticoagulant treatment was definitely demonstrated.

Remarkable as these anticoagulants have proved to be, they are not a sure cure for heart attack. Medical science makes no such claims. Nevertheless, they tend to prevent one of the most dreaded complications of heart attack—the occurrence of a second heart attack—by reducing the tendency of the blood to clot.

Anticoagulants are not needed in every case. So if your doctor does not give you an anticoagulant, don't think you're not receiving the most up-to-date treatment. Many patients do not need them at all. If the attack is rather light and, in the physician's careful judgment, there is hardly any danger of further clotting, neither of these anticoagulant drugs are used. Even though the possibility of bleeding as a side-effect has been practically eliminated today, no useful purpose would be served by the use of anticoagulants if the patient can recover just as well without them.

Of course, the clotting time must not be reduced too greatly, in order to avoid the possibility of bleeding. For this reason patients who are being treated with anticoagulants are watched closely. At least once a day, or as often as the physician deems necessary, blood is taken and sent to the laboratory to determine the clotting time. Clotting time can be accurately measured, and the patient receives only as much of the medication as can be given safely. If there should be even the slightest sign of minute bleeding, it can be checked very effectively within three to six hours by the use of Vitamin K.

Lately, other anticoagulant preparations have been developed that are said to be safer and yet equally effective. Investigators, among them Dr. Link himself, who developed one of these new preparations in his laboratory, are highly enthusiastic about them. Although it is still too soon to judge their advantages over the original drugs, one important improvement is that the action of these newer preparations is much more rapid, so that the expensive heparin very likely will no longer be needed.

Long-Range Use of Anticoagulants

Use of the anticoagulants during the acute stage of a heart attack represents the most remarkable modern advance in medical treatment. However, once the imminent danger is eliminated, the possibility still remains that, much later, a new clot may be formed in some other part of the coronary artery that similarly had been narrowed down. A new heart attack may occur months or years afterwards. Since the introduction of anticoagulant drugs in treating the acute phase of heart attack to prevent enlarging of the original blood clot, many specialists continued to prescribe anticoagulants for some patients even after the acute phase was over, but in much smaller doses.

As long as the patient is taking an anticoagulant drug, the chemistry of his blood is changed so that it will not clot easily. The drug will have no effect on the fatty deposits that have accumulated in the lining of the coronary artery here and there. But because of the presence of the anticoagulant, the blood remains fluid and does not clot so readily as it flows through these roughened spots. This new kind of long-range use of anticoagulants has already been tried out on a sufficient number of patients to allow us to form an opinion as to whether it can prevent new heart attacks.

At the Second World Congress of Cardiology held in Washington, D. C., in September, 1954, investigators reported their findings on 1,100 patients who had been treated with anticoagulants for a long time, and who were observed for periods ranging from six months to eight years. The outcome was then compared with that of 500 patients who had had a heart attack but had not received anticoagulants. The conclusion of these investigators was that anticoagulants definitely prevented the formation of fresh thrombi and, in general, prolonged life expectancy considerably. Aside from this directly beneficial effect, anginal pain in patients who had recovered from the acute attack almost always ceased after anticoagulant treatment was instituted.

In another study made in South Africa, 82 patients who received anticoagulants were compared with 88 patients who did not. For the anticoagulant treatment, these doctors selected patients who had suffered more than one heart attack and who, generally, were more seriously ill. The period of observation ranged from one to six years. Their findings once more proved the efficiency of anticoagulants. Mortality for the group who did not receive anticoagulants was 33 per cent, while for those who did receive anticoagulants, and who were more seriously ill, the mortality was only slightly over 7 per cent, which represented more than a four-fold reduction. In the treated group there were only seven cases of a fresh attack, while in the control group 24 suffered further attacks.

The treatment is especially effective in patients who had suffered more than one heart attack during the course of years. As a number of further studies have shown, the mortality rate of those who had suffered more than one heart attack was only a fifth of that of untreated patients.

Anticoagulants, together with other modern methods, have reduced the death rate in the early phases of a heart attack so greatly that the vast majority recover from the initial attack. And this means not only that the heart itself is mended but, on the average, in one to four months after leaving the hospital the great majority will be able to resume a normal life. With proper self-care, these persons will be able to return to their former occupation, a large proportion of them without the slightest restriction of activity.

As a matter of fact, persons who recover from the initial attack are already on the way to recovery. But after you leave the hospital, how well you'll be able to adjust to a new way of life and achieve complete rehabilitation will largely depend on you.

Dr. L. S. Kubie, in an important paper read at a session of

the New York Academy of Medicine, described four phases in the process of recovery:

1. Initial shock.
2. Stage of appreciation of the full extent of disability.
3. Recovery from the lure of hospital care.
4. The stage of facing independent, unsupported, competitive life.

We shall now consider the third phase, the days and weeks after leaving the hospital.

8

Convalescence

AFTER the average patient has overcome the initial shock and fear of imminent death, he becomes somewhat calmed down. With each succeeding day he gains a little more confidence. Unless he is of an unusually anxious type, he becomes increasingly sure he is going to recover. Of course, the person who is stable, not easily ruffled by life situations, will take his condition more calmly than the individual who is fearful and apprehensive by nature. The overactive, ambitious, and driving type of person will be impatient, resentful of any restriction, and the physician will have some difficulty in keeping him in the hospital.

But whatever their psychological make-up, most persons, by placing their fate entirely in the hands of the physician, can at least relegate to the back of their minds the overwhelming fear of death. Perhaps because of an unrecognized or unadmitted desire to escape personal responsibility, or because it is a subconscious defense mechanism, as long as the patient is in the hospital under the constant supervision and care of doctor and nurses, he feels that nothing can possibly happen to him. His ailment does not seem to him any more serious than the ailments of other patients in the hospital. He is sure he will get over it, just as do the patients with appendicitis or pneumonia, who leave the hospital every day.

However, as soon as he gets home from the hospital, the full impact of his condition strikes him suddenly. For the first time he becomes fully aware that there is something wrong with his heart. He becomes panicky, anxious, alarmed, or over-depressed, picturing himself as a chronic invalid, no longer able to support himself or his family.

A few years ago the Cleveland Work Classification Clinic reported that emotional factors presented the greatest difficulties in nearly one-half of former heart attack victims who were examined for re-employment. Some of these individuals had been rather fearful, anxious, and tense before their heart attack. But even in those who were by psychological make-up more stable, the occurrence of heart attack brought on fear, anxiety, and depression.

All this unreasoning fear and depression can invariably be traced back to a complete misconception by the average person of what heart attack actually means. Correction of such a popular misconception is urgent, and not only to ease the mind of persons who at one time or other have suffered a heart attack. Studies carried out more than two decades ago have shown that emotions definitely have a direct effect on the work of the heart. More recently, delicate direct measurements on the work of the human heart have shown that emotions markedly increase the work of even the normal heart. Such an extra burden on an already somewhat impaired heart is dangerous.

Such unreasonable fear has an equally and perhaps even more serious drawback for the person who has just come home from the hospital. What he actually should do is to become gradually more active, to move about more freely, and in general to purposefully increase the burden he places on his heart. Yet overfearful patients avoid any activity at all. No amount of persuasion by the doctor will be able to convince them that they need work just as much as they needed rest immediately after the heart attack.

Dismiss at once from your mind the popular idea that every person who has had a heart attack will be, at least to some extent, incapacitated for the rest of his life. Nothing could be further from the truth.

And do not think for a moment that a complete recovery is an almost miraculous rarity. Investigators during the past two decades have published a number of large-scale studies that reported the subsequent fate of victims of a heart attack.

The Odds Are in Your Favor

The most recent as well as the most detailed follow-up study of how the average person fares after a heart attack was made by Dr. Arthur M. Master and his fellow-workers. This paper should be sufficient to dispel the exaggerated fear, the pessimism, and the hopelessness with which most heart attack victims contemplate their future.

For nearly three decades Dr. Master and his co-workers followed the subsequent fate of 500 patients, 415 men and 85 women. The period of observation for the entire group averaged six and a half years, but for none of them less than one year, so that enough time elapsed for the experimenters to tell how the patient had fared. Quite a number of these patients had had their heart attack much earlier than the average of six and a half years. Among the latter was a physician, in perfect health and engaged in active practice with practically no restriction of activities, who had had a heart attack twenty-nine years prior to the publication of this study. The average age of these 500 persons at the time they suffered the heart attack was slightly over fifty-three years.

Each of these patients was repeatedly examined during the course of this study. The investigators noted whether they had any difficulties or not, and, if so, to what extent; how well they were able to engage in ordinary activities; the kind of work they were engaged in; and in general how they compared with persons who had never had a heart attack. In addition, every one of them was subjected to complete physical examination, including electrocardiogram, X-ray studies, blood pressure—in short, everything to enable these physicians to gain a complete picture of the condition of the heart. According to the degree of recovery, the investigators divided these patients into four groups:

	Number	%

GROUP 1:
Persons who never experienced any pain, difficulty in breathing, or the slightest weakness, had no need whatsoever to curtail any of their activities, and who were fully capable of resuming their former occupation. In short, their recovery was so complete that repeated medical examination failed to reveal any evidence of a previous heart attack. — 209 — 41.8

GROUP 2:
Persons who experienced some mild pain occasionally, but only after unusual exertion or great emotional upset. Nevertheless, they had no need to restrict their activities to any appreciable degree and were certainly fit to resume their former occupation. — 213 — 42.6

GROUP 3:
Persons who experienced moderate chest pain on exertion and who complained of feeling weak from time to time. Despite these difficulties, a number of these patients, as judged by the doctors, were able to do partial work, and a surprising number could do full time work. — 50 — 10.0

GROUP 4:
Persons who had rather severe chest pains, evidenced some signs of heart failure, and needed to restrict their activities to a much greater extent. Nevertheless, not every one of these could be classified as a heart cripple. Two of this group, both of them executives, continued to work at least part time. — 28 — 5.6

This study, then, revealed that four out of every five persons made either a complete or a highly satisfactory recovery, judged by any standards. Only a few more than 5 per cent were incapacitated to a more serious extent.

Other large-scale studies show that anywhere from 75 to 85 per cent of all persons who have suffered a heart attack are able to perform gainful work, and almost always in the same kind of occupation they had been engaged in prior to the attack.

The Gillette Safety Razor Company in Boston found that the average employee who had completely recovered from a heart attack, if placed properly, is not only productive but actually rates somewhat higher than others. One reason is that such an employee is more experienced and more skillful because of the years he has spent with the company. Such a person has a greater incentive to prove himself as capable as the other employees.

It is highly important for you, while recovering from a heart attack, to assume a much more realistic attitude about your chances of going back to work again. A number of studies involving accurate measurements have shown that physical activity following a heart attack speeds up the complete recovery of a damaged heart. Recently, Dr. R. W. Eckstein reported to the Scientific Session of the American Heart Association that in dogs whose coronary artery has been greatly narrowed by artificial means, collateral circulation appeared much sooner and was far more efficient if the dogs had undergone a rigorous schedule of exercise.

If you believe that your heart has become so weakened by the heart attack that it will never be nearly so strong as it was before, you'll be likely to be too timid and overcautious, avoiding even the slightest effort. *This is exactly the opposite of what you should do.* Gradually increased physical activity, far from being harmful, will help the heart regain its tone so that it can respond more readily to any extra burden placed upon it. Large-scale studies have shown that physically active patients live longer and are less likely to suffer a second heart attack than persons who remain completely inactive.

Getting Ready for Work

The average person will be able to return to work after spending from one to three months at home following his release from the hospital. This means that you can count on getting back on the job from three to six months after your heart attack. A few patients who have an extremely mild attack may do so even much sooner, and extremely few will require more than six months. You should consider this period at home as a preparation for resuming full activity. Naturally, the first three weeks or so at the job you'll take it rather easy until you feel completely fit.

The patient who accepts his heart attack as simply an episode, a bout of illness certainly far less serious than many others, a temporary interruption of his usual activities, will have the proper motivation to help his own recovery to the fullest extent.

The physician will outline the general schedule to be followed during convalescence according to the needs of the individual. As a rule, the average patient is permitted to get out of bed in the morning of the first day of the seventh week and to sit in a chair for fifteen minutes, and for the same length of time in the afternoon. For the next three days he is allowed to sit up fifteen minutes more than the day before, so that on the fourth day he can be up for a full hour, morning and afternoon. After this he should add half an hour each time.

However, you will be allowed to take only a few steps in the room until the end of the seventh week. By that time you can walk around the room a little more each day. When the allotted time to sit in the chair reaches four hours in the morning and four in the afternoon, it will be a good idea to arrange your schedule so that you get up with leisure in the morning, stay up until lunch time, and then take a rest in bed for two hours in the afternoon. After this you can stay up again until dinnertime.

In general, the physician will emphasize what you can do rather than what you cannot do. As important as rest has been during the first six weeks, an ever-increasing activity afterward without undue fear is exactly as important for full recovery, or perhaps even more so.

Dr. Herman K. Hellerstein, an authority in the field of rehabilitation of the heart attack victim, goes so far as to state that "the patient should be allowed to increase his activities to the point of slight discomfort."

And he adds significantly: "The desire to return to work should be nurtured by increasing the number of contacts with the outside world and helping the patient formulate work plans."

How Much Can You Do?

No doubt you have been warned by well-meaning friends scrupulously to avoid stairs. As a matter of fact, some persons sell their homes and buy a ranch-type house with one floor. Or at least they move to a first-floor apartment.

The advice to avoid stairs certainly seems reasonable. But just how much truth is there in it? A few years ago Dr. J. A. L. Mathers and his co-workers went to the trouble of finding out by actual measurements what the facts are. They had both healthy men and those on the way to recovery walk up and down steps, and then they measured the work involved in it. These measurements revealed that climbing steps increased the work of the heart only to a slight degree, certainly within the ability of even a somewhat damaged heart. A really surprising finding was that going up the steps imposed no more work on the heart than coming down. The amount of work required in either direction was only slightly greater than walking an equal distance on level ground.

Many heart specialists, far from telling their patients to avoid steps altogether, advise them, after gaining a little more strength, to go up and down one flight of stairs once a day for a few days, then several times a day, at first slowly, until they are able to walk up and down at a normal pace.

But climbing steps is not the only activity the average patient avoids unnecessarily. They are as a rule too timid about many activities that, in fact, do not require too much energy. Fortunately, today we don't need to guess what you can do and what you should postpone for a while at least. Scientists have accurately measured the amount of work involved in ordinary home activities, as well as in the various jobs in office, factory, or any other kind of occupation.

Energy Costs of Various Activities

The most widely used and at the same time the most accurate method of comparing the various activities is by measuring how much they cost in terms of energy expenditure. When a person is at complete rest, his body burns up approximately one calorie every minute. This is the minimum expenditure needed for the vital functions of the body. Therefore, the minimum, or as it is called, basal, energy expenditure is used as a yardstick.

When you start to drive your car you give it more gas; that is, your car will need more fuel than when the motor is idling. The faster you drive, the more gas you will need. It is the same with the human body. When you do anything, your body will need more energy than it does when you are at complete rest. The more energy needed, the harder the heart has to pump to supply the necessary blood for the entire body.

Dr. Edward E. Gordon, Director of the Department of Physical Medicine of Michael Reese Hospital, prepared a list of what different kinds of self-care activities cost in terms of energy expenditure.

TABLE 1

COST OF SELF-CARE ACTIVITIES IN CALORIES PER MINUTE

Activity	Cal./min.	Activity	Cal./min.
Rest—supine	1.0	Dressing, undressing	2.3
Sitting	1.2	Washing, hand, face	2.5
Standing, relaxed	1.4	Beside commode	3.6
Eating	1.4	Walking (2.5 mph)	3.6
Conversation	1.4	Showering	4.2
Using bedpan	4.7	Walking downstairs	5.2

This means that by simply sitting up you add 20 per cent to the work of the heart as compared with the resting state, 40 per cent more while eating, and when you walk downstairs the heart must work five times as hard.

So it would seem that even ordinary daily activities place a good deal of burden on the heart. Yet these requirements are well within the capacity of the heart without its being overloaded.

The ability of the human heart to perform is truly astonishing. Scientists measured the energy expenditure of champion athletes during a two-mile run or in competitive skiing. They found that during the duration of the race these champion athletes maintained an energy expenditure of 26.5 calories per minute, that is, their heart worked more than 26 times harder than when at rest. Other scientists measured the energy expenditure of a number of healthy men who were not trained for athletic activities. These men were capable of increasing the per minute expenditure up to 14 calories.

The work the heart must perform during the race seems tremendous. And remember, the career of the athlete extends to many years, during which, even when he is not engaged in contest, he must train strenuously. Yet this heightened activity over many years does not damage his heart at all.

Not so many years ago, even doctors spoke of "athlete's heart." Today we know there is no such thing. If anything, an athlete's heart may be in better condition precisely because of those years engaged in athletic activities. Furthermore, it has been definitely shown that no amount of work can possibly damage a normal heart.

How much energy do you yourself actually exert when you are engaged in ordinary recreational activities?

The next table, using the same yardstick of calorie expenditure per minute, shows the energy cost of various recreational activities.

TABLE 2

COST OF RECREATIONAL ACTIVITIES IN CALORIES PER MINUTE

Activity	Cal./min.	Activity	Cal./min.
Painting	2.0	Swimming (20 yd. min.)	5.0
Playing piano	2.5	Dancing	5.5
Driving car	2.8	Gardening	5.6
Canoeing (2.5 mph)	3.0	Trotting horse	8.0
Horseback riding (slow)	3.0	Spading	8.6
Volley ball	3.5	Skiing	9.9
Bowling	4.4	Squash	10.2
Golfing	5.0	Cycling (13 mph)	11.0

Naturally, you wouldn't be tempted shortly after a heart attack to go skiing or to do any spading, or even to drive a car, although the latter activity uses even less energy than taking a shower. Nevertheless, this will serve as a guide to what kind of recreation you can have later on, after you have returned to your job and have regained your full strength.

How much energy does the average person use up in home activities and recreation? Actual measurements have shown that the eight waking hours he spends away from his job require an average of three calories per minute.

For the woman, the following table shows how much various household activities cost in terms of energy expenditure.

TABLE 3

COST OF VARIOUS HOUSEHOLD TASKS IN CALORIES PER MINUTE

Activity	Cal./min.	Activity	Cal./min.
Hand sewing	1.4	Scrubbing floors	3.6
Sweeping floor	1.7	Cleaning windows	3.7
Machine sewing	1.8	Making beds	3.9
Polishing	2.4	Ironing, standing	4.2
Peeling potatoes	2.9	Mopping	4.2
Scrubbing, standing	2.9	Wringing by hand	4.4
Washing small clothes	3.0	Hanging wash	4.5
Kneading dough	3.3	Beating carpets	4.9

The energy costs of some of these household chores will no doubt surprise you, for many of them require far less expenditure of energy than most people imagine. But those that are likely to impose too great a burden on the heart should be avoided at first and then resumed slowly and cautiously as you gradually build up your over-all fitness.

You can see from this table that when you are ironing, for example, your heart will have to work four times as hard as when you are resting. So during the early phases of recovery, at least, you should avoid doing any ironing or any other of the chores requiring comparatively high expenditure of energy. Even those needing less energy should be carried out with leisure and with frequent rest. As your strength returns you will be able to do a little more each day, and so gradually condition yourself for the heavier chores.

Training

Everyone appreciates the importance of training for athletes. You certainly don't expect a heavyweight champion to step into the ring for a 15-round championship fight after he has been out of training for six months or more. Your favorite pitcher won't be in midseason form the day he reports for spring training. What expert training does is to bring to razor edge the athlete's natural ability, which was dormant as long as he was not using it to the utmost.

The human heart, just like the untrained athlete, must be given the opportunity to develop to its fullest capacity. The heart has a far greater potential capacity for work than it will ever be called upon to use, even the heart that has been damaged by a heart attack.

As you can see in Table 1, walking requires only a moderate amount of energy expenditure. Walking, then, is one of the most efficient ways of self-training. Besides being easy on the heart, walking relieves boredom from being largely confined to a room. And boredom helps to induce anxiety, which places a far greater burden on the heart than does the pleasant pastime of walking.

One of the best ways you can judge how well you are progressing is to keep a daily record of how far you can walk without getting tired or short of breath. The minute you get the least bit tired or have a tight feeling in your chest, stop at once and rest for a minute or two. You should be able to walk a little more each day without getting tired.

The amount of work you place on your heart when you are walking does not depend so much on how fast you walk as it does on the nature of the ground. Walking uphill imposes far more work on the heart than walking at the same pace on level ground. The figure on page 90 illustrates how much harder the heart has to work when you walk uphill.

You can see from this illustration that a person walking on level ground expends four calories per minute compared to 5.5

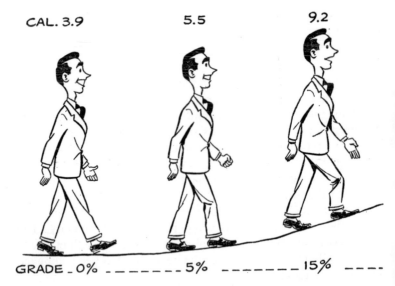

CAL. 3.9   5.5   9.2

GRADE _ 0% _ _ _ _ _ _ _ 5% _ _ _ _ _ _ _ 15% _ _ _ _

Figure 5. CALORIE EXPENDITURE PER MINUTE IN WALKING UP-
HILL AT 2.5 MPH. (After Edward E. Gordon, M.D., "The Ex-
penditure of Energy in Health and in Disease," *Medical Science,*
January, 1958)

calories per minute when walking up a 5 per cent grade, and
nine calories per minute up a 15 per cent grade. You can readily
see that in the latter instance the heart will have to work twice
as hard as on level ground. For this reason, persons who are
subject to anginal attacks or whose heart reserve is not sufficient
for suddenly increased demands should avoid walking uphill,
and especially in cold and windy weather.

Again, how far a person can walk without distress depends a
good deal on how heavy he is. Scientists measured the energy
expenditure of persons of various weights walking on level
ground, and found that the heavier a person is the greater will
be the stress imposed on his heart. For example, a man weighing 200 pounds imposes about 25 per cent more work on his
heart than a man of 140 pounds performing the same task. So
it is obvious that overweight is an added handicap to a heart

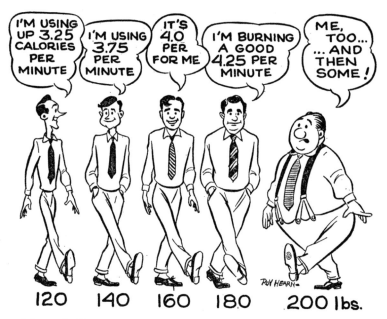

Figure 6. CALORIE COST WITH INCREASE IN WEIGHT, WALKING AT 2.5 MPH.

that has already been somewhat damaged. This is one more reason why the person recovering from a heart attack should keep his weight down.

As the person is gradually recovering from a heart attack he will be able to increase his activities without becoming unduly tired. And in this way he gains increasing confidence in himself. But the best indication that he is well on the road to recovery is when he asks the doctor about smoking and, perhaps even more importantly, when he wants to find out when he will be allowed to resume sex relations.

9

Tobacco, Alcohol and Sex

IT WOULD hardly be an exaggeration to say that no medical research has been more widely publicized and better known to the general public than that relating to cigarette smoking and lung cancer.

Now, in respect to cigarette smoking and heart attack, there are two questions to which you'd like to have an answer. The first is whether or not long-continued smoking can originate or aggravate changes in the coronary arteries to such an extent that it will eventually lead to heart attack.

The second is whether or not smoking is harmful to you if you have already had a heart attack.

These two questions are not necessarily the same. It is conceivable that smoking may have nothing to do with deterioration of the coronary artery and yet may have a deleterious effect on an already diseased coronary.

Can Smoking Induce Coronary Artery Changes?

As to the first question, namely, whether or not smoking can lead to coronary heart disease, one thing should be made clear in the beginning. In contrast to the enormous amount of research work done in the field of lung cancer, studies in regard to the connection of smoking and development of coronary disease are surprisingly few. Furthermore, the evidence is exclusively of a statistical nature.

The most impressive of such statistical evidence is furnished by a study made by the American Cancer Society. In the first five months of 1952, volunteer interviewers for the Cancer Society obtained the smoking history of nearly 200,000 men and women, that is, whether they smoked or not, and if they did, how much and what kind of tobacco they used. After a lapse of 18 months, the same interviewers checked the subsequent fate of nearly every one of those originally interviewed.

This study was primarily concerned with the possible connection of cigarette smoking and lung cancer. It was almost as a second thought that it was extended to deaths from coronary heart disease. Here we are concerned only with these findings.

During this 18-month period a number of persons originally interviewed for the study died. The interviewers, then, obtained the cause of death in nearly all of these cases—4,710, to be exact. According to the death certificates, nearly half of these had died from coronary heart disease.

After tabulating deaths from coronary heart disease according to age groups, investigators found that in the age group of fifty to sixty-four the death rate was 95 per cent higher among smokers than among non-smokers. However, rather curiously, in the age group between sixty-four and sixty-nine the coronary death rate was found to be only 15 per cent higher for smokers than for non-smokers.

This fact alone should make us stop to ask some pertinent questions. An older person, naturally, has smoked for a considerably longer time than a younger one. If smoking has any deleterious effect on the coronary artery, the difference in death rate between smokers and non-smokers should be expected to be higher among older than among younger persons. But according to these statistics, the opposite was true. The difference was smaller among older than among younger persons.

Nevertheless, these statistics show that, in general, the death rate from coronary disease is higher among smokers than among non-smokers. But before we accept this as a valid conclusion, we must ask ourselves some questions.

The first rule of all statistical studies is that the number included must be large enough and taken at random, and, furthermore, without a preconceived idea, in order to be applicable to the entire group, in this case the general population above a certain age.

The American Cancer Society's study included a large number of deaths from coronary disease. Furthermore, it is in no sense selective. In that regard it is a fair sample, applicable to the general population. However, this numerically large study is open to serious question on another count: Do these figures cover actual deaths from heart attack?

All medical scientists agree that the only way the cause of death from heart attack can be positively established is by autopsy. Yet of the death certificates used in this study, the vast majority were made out without an autopsy record. What proportion of these deaths was due to something else than the one shown on the death certificate, no one knows. For this reason, data obtained from death certificates cannot be used in a scientific work. As Dr. Harry S. N. Greene, Chairman of the Department of Pathology of Yale University, in connection with another disease, but even more applicable to death from heart attack, stated: ". . . statistics based on death certificates are practically valueless in this respect, and the only material suitable for analysis is that derived from . . . autopsy reports."

But this is not the only consideration that presents extreme difficulty in trying to decide from statistics alone the possible role of smoking in causing coronary heart disease.

Smoking and Coronary Patients

There have been a few studies made in the past two decades regarding the smoking habits of coronary patients. These are highly accurate, since the diagnosis in each case had been established definitely. But even a glance at these statistics

brings out one glaring fact that has been consistently ignored—
that in the great majority of heart attack victims, smoking
could not possibly have played any role, for the simple reason
that these persons either did not smoke at all or smoked only
moderately.

One study, for example, showed that 13 per cent of persons
with coronary disease were heavy smokers. The implicit fact
that 87 per cent were non-smokers or at least not heavy users
of tobacco is conveniently forgotten. If smoking could bring
on heart disease, an entirely legitimate question would be: Why
did those 87 per cent of non-smokers develop coronary heart
disease?

This objection may, of course, be countered by saying that
the 13 per cent were especially susceptible to tobacco. Or perhaps that tobacco must have been only a contributing cause.
Or that persons can develop coronary disease from other causes.
It may be so for all we know. However, there is nothing whatsoever in the figures themselves that would justify such assumptions.

Nevertheless, other studies, again based on statistics, would
make such assumptions extremely dubious, to say the least.

In this study, heavy smokers constituted 13 per cent of the
entire group treated by that physician. Another physician reported that among his patients 17 per cent were heavy smokers. Still another found that 24.4 per cent of his patients were
heavy smokers. And a fourth physician reported that the heavy
smokers constituted 50 per cent of his coronary patients. All
these patients were Americans who had suffered a heart attack
during the past two decades.

It is obvious that groups of persons with the same background, the same make-up, and the same general habits could
not possibly differ so tremendously as to susceptibility to
smoking.

But there is still another question. Does smoking inevitably
lead to coronary disease? For the answer to this, we must turn
to a very recent Swiss study of 149 men over the age of fifty, including practically an equal number of healthy persons and

coronary patients. It was found that 45 per cent of the coronary group were heavy smokers. However, 28.5 per cent of the healthy men also smoked habitually more than 20 cigarettes a day.

Although the percentage among coronary patients was definitely higher, the fact remains that 28.5 per cent of heavy smokers did not develop coronary disease. The natural question would be: Why didn't that 28.5 per cent develop coronary heart disease?

The answer could be that, given enough time, the 28.5 per cent would also develop coronary disease. That would be entirely beside the point, however, for if we are trying to answer a question by statistical methods we must stick to the data that we actually have and not indulge in sheer speculation. Whether these men will or will not develop coronary disease must be left to the future, but it cannot be considered here.

So, the answer to whether excessive smoking inevitably leads to coronary disease must, at least according to these statistics, be an emphatic no.

Finally, one more recent study should be mentioned. As a part of a study, Dr. Menard R. Gertler and Dr. Paul Dudley White obtained the accurate history of 90 men under forty with coronary heart disease, and of 139 perfectly healthy males of corresponding age, in regard to their smoking habits. On the basis of their statistical analysis, these doctors stated that the difference in the two groups of smokers and non-smokers was so small as to be almost negligible. In other words, cigarette smoking apparently plays no role in development of coronary artery disease.

Is Smoking Injurious After a Heart Attack?

Now we turn to the second question proposed at the beginning of this chapter: Will smoking be harmful for a person who has had a heart attack?

This is a question of immediate interest to you. After all, very few persons would be willing to give up a pleasant habit even if they were fully convinced it *might,* in the distant future, cause definite injury to their coronaries. But if they were told after they had a heart attack that smoking is *definitely* harmful to them, they would at least be likely to make an effort to quit.

If you have never smoked, or if you quit some time ago, the question of whether tobacco does or does not harm the heart is of no interest to you. Certainly, no one has as yet suggested that you start smoking to improve your condition. However, if you are a confirmed smoker, and the chances are that you are, the situation is far different. To give up smoking is a decision so extremely difficult for most persons that only a very convincing reason will induce them to give it a trial. Naturally, a confirmed smoker wants to know what science has to say in this regard, and what the actual score is, for and against.

There is no longer any doubt that smoking cigarettes can affect the circulatory system. However, it is equally certain that it does not affect every individual to the same degree. In some persons the effect is rather pronounced, in others it is very slight, and in still others there is no effect at all.

In what way does smoking affect the circulatory system? Without marshalling tiresome figures, it may be stated that smoking cigarettes is capable of increasing the pulse rate and of raising blood pressure to some extent.

Precise and accurate experiments on the immediate effect of smoking have shown unequivocally that even one cigarette can produce constriction of the capillaries (the finest blood vessels) of the skin. But again, not in every person. Furthermore, the degree of constriction differs considerably from individual to individual. The effect, of course, wears off in a short time.

From this undoubted effect of tobacco on the capillaries of the skin, some investigators assume that it must have the same effect on the coronary artery itself—that is, constrict it. No doubt you have heard one kind of argument in trying to convince you that smoking is bad for the heart. This argument is that since tobacco is a constrictor of the blood vessels it would naturally constrict the coronary artery, the last thing you would want to do if you've had a heart attack. The reasoning is very logical and convincing to everybody. *The only trouble is that it is absolutely untrue.*

Nicotine constricts the capillaries of the skin, but it has no effect whatsoever on the coronary. The mechanisms that regulate the changes in the caliber of the capillaries of the skin are entirely different from those regulating the changes in the larger arteries, including the coronary. We know, for example, that a chemical substance produced by the body narrows down considerably the capillaries of the skin, but the same substance dilates the deeper arteries of the body.

Dr. Henry I. Russek, who with his co-workers carried out extensive experimental studies on the effects of nicotine, states that smoking does not constitute "a direct danger to the patient with coronary artery disease through the medium of coronary vasoconstriction (narrowing)."

Although nicotine has no effect whatever on the coronary artery itself, there is some scientific evidence that small amounts of tobacco or nicotine actually increase the flow of blood in the coronary, apparently without changing its caliber.

But do not take this latter finding as an encouragement to smoke even more cigarettes than you did before. Nicotine, but again not invariably and not in every person, may change the condition of the heart muscle itself. And such changes can be detected by means of the electrocardiogram and ballistogram.

Persons who have recovered from a heart attack are more likely than healthy persons to show changes in their electrocardiogram and ballistogram tracings after smoking. These changes may be wholly insignificant, or so slight as to indicate no added burden to the heart. However, in some individuals who are presumably more susceptible to nicotine the effect may be marked and actually detrimental to health. Physicians have known for a long time that there are some individuals in whom smoking induces severe pain resembling true angina. That such symptoms are directly due to tobacco is shown by the fact that they promptly disappear when smoking is discontinued.

All this, then, demonstrates conclusively that some persons are highly susceptible to the effect of smoking. Needless to say, such persons should not smoke at all.

But the question is: How can we tell who belongs in this category? One way, of course, would be to carry out tests on everyone who has had a heart attack, but this is obviously impracticable. The easiest way is for each individual to test himself. If you develop chest pain or other disturbing symptoms after smoking, and if these symptoms disappear when you stop smoking, you can decide for yourelf that smoking is not for you.

If the above discussion leaves you in the position of the gambler who decides the next step by a flip of the coin, remember that everything in life involves a certain amount of gamble. But we must be very emphatic on one point: No gamble must be permitted during the acute phase of a heart attack. Even one cigarette imposes an extra burden on the heart, no matter how slight. Since during this period absolute rest must be obtained, the patient must not be allowed to smoke at all.

The Case for Cigarettes

The arguments of those who defend smoking say that it soothes jagged nerves, is calming for the mind, and affords relaxation. This is undeniably true, and is another reason why a person should not be deprived of the little pleasures of life without compelling reasons.

There is still another consideration that the physican takes into account in deciding whether he should or should not allow his patients to smoke. A man who is recovering from a heart attack and is well on the way to resuming useful work needs a good deal of encouragement to restore his self-confidence. If he is told at every turn that he must not do this and must not do that, he cannot help thinking that he is still a very sick person and that he must watch every step very carefully. In retraining the patient after the acute phase of the heart attack is over, he should be told what he is allowed to do rather than what he cannot do.

A person who quits smoking usually starts to eat candy in order to relieve that aching void created by giving up cigarettes. Furthermore, many persons who smoke a good deal have a somewhat diminished appetite for food, possibly because the taste buds in the tongue are somewhat deadened. When they stop smoking, the sense of taste returns. Consequently, both because of an improved sense of taste, and also for psychological reasons, the average person who gives up cigarettes starts to eat to excess.

There is not the slightest doubt among the greatest authorities that overweight constitutes a definite and real hazard for the person who has recovered from a heart attack.

Coffee and Tea

Many persons are afraid to drink coffee or tea if they have had a heart attack, in the belief that these beverages are too stimulating and add to the burden of the heart. It is true that if you drink too many cups of coffee or tea your heart is likely to pound too fast. But this is also true for healthy persons as well as cardiacs. The fact is, however, that neither of these beverages, if used in moderation, imposes any burden on the heart. As a matter of fact, they are actually beneficial. In the morning, a cup of coffee helps to brighten up the mind and give more zest for the day's tasks ahead. Later in the day an occasional cup of coffee is wonderfully refreshing—a coffee break.

As a matter of fact, doctors used to prescribe the active ingredient of coffee and tea in a form of drug in treating heart attack. At that time it was believed that this drug dilates the coronary blood vessels and thus increases the blood supply to the heart. Later, however, it was found that neither this drug nor coffee and tea have the effect of dilating the coronary arteries.

While coffee and tea certainly have no curative value, they definitely are not harmful in moderation, and they may actually be beneficial for other reasons. Naturally, a cup of coffee late in the evening may have the effect of preventing your falling asleep. If coffee does this to you, you should avoid it a few hours before retiring. This is practically the only precaution you have to observe in regard to coffee and tea.

Alcohol

For a long time alcohol had the reputation, even among physicians, of being able to dilate the coronary arteries and so increase the flow of blood through them. We know now, however, that alcohol in any form has no such effect. Nevertheless, if not as a dilator of the coronary, alcohol does have a beneficial effect for the person recovering from a heart attack. Alcohol has a soothing effect on the nerves, enabling the person to relax. In addition, it is a mild pain killer.

During the period of convalescence, an occasional drink will be beneficial, provided, of course, you have previously been in the habit of taking a drink from time to time. Aside from its obvious soothing effects, the knowledge that a patient is allowed to use alcoholic beverages in moderation will add a good deal to his self-confidence. Just as with the smoker, a usually vigorous and self-sufficient man will feel hemmed in and frustrated by too many taboos and don'ts. After complete recovery, of course, there is no reason whatever for him to refrain from moderate drinking.

Alcohol used to excess is another thing. In the first place, intoxication may place too much burden on the heart. A man who is slightly high and feels wonderful doesn't realize that his breathing rate is increased, his heart speeds up, and so do the burning-up processes of the entire body.

The worst and perhaps a potentially dangerous thing is that, with a few too many drinks under his belt, a man may be tempted to do too much. As a rule, he will overestimate his strength, and the result is that he becomes boisterous in more ways than one. Such overactivity may be dangerous for his heart.

The alcoholic who has suffered a heart attack presents an

entirely different problem, one that does not primarily concern us here. Trying to scare the alcoholic away from the bottle by telling him how it will eventually harm his health, however, is of no help whatsoever.

The ability of the alcoholic to find excuses is truly remarkable. If he has had a heart attack he is bound to explain that now he really needs alcohol, as it is beneficial for his coronaries. It would be useless to try to tell him that alcohol has no such effect. It would serve a more useful purpose if a sympathetic doctor, without any attempt to condemn him on moral grounds, could point out to him that every time he gets drunk he is overloading his heart to such an extent that sooner or later it is bound to break down completely.

It can also happen that a moderate drinker, after suffering a heart attack, becomes so despondent and assumes such a devil-may-care attitude that he becomes a drunkard. Experts on alcoholism know that some kind of tragedy, given a certain type of personality, may lead a person to alcoholism.

If such a person fully realizes that a heart attack in most cases does not mean that his active days are over and, above all, if he does not regard his heart attack as an irreparable tragedy, he will take a more cheerful attitude and so will be less likely to find solace in the bottle.

For the majority of drinkers, who can take it or leave it, alcohol is no problem. Nevertheless, even for those who drink moderately, there is something that should be taken into consideration—the matter of calories. If you like a bottle of beer occasionally, remember that it contains around 110 calories, and a shot of whiskey somewhere around 90 calories. If you have to watch your calories, don't forget to include this in your dietary budget. Beer also contains a small amount of salt, so if you're on a low salt diet, remember to take this into consideration also.

Sex Life

When a man is suddenly stricken with a heart attack and is flat on his back, sex will probably be the farthest thing from his mind. Even during convalescence, especially since most of the victims are middle-aged, sex is usually not an urgent problem. But when the patient is well on the road to recovery and begins to think in terms of resuming life where he left off, the question of sex becomes more important.

Not so long ago a man recovering from a heart attack was much too embarrassed to ask his physician whether he would be allowed to indulge in sexual activities. Even more often, such a man wouldn't even bother to ask, for he would take it for granted that sexual activity would impose so much strain on his weakened heart that he could not resume that part of his life for many months or even years. Indeed, only a few years ago his physician would probably have confirmed his fear. He would have told him that the excitement and heightened tension, resulting in rise in blood pressure and sudden strain on his heart, would involve such a tremendous risk that the best thing would be for him to forget all about sex.

Today, the physician, far from prohibiting it, will actually prescribe sex for him. True, the rise in blood pressure, the quickening of the pulse, the enhanced labor of the heart, is real and measurable. However, such strain is well within the reserves of the heart to sustain. Even more importantly, normal sex life undoubtedly represents the most satisfactory means for release of inner tension. Furthermore, the complete emotional and physical relaxation that comes from marital relations will help prevent the sense of frustration that overly restricted activity in any sphere will invariably produce.

To some men, sex is a means of expressing their sense of mastery; to others it is a reassurance of virility; and in not a few, a subconsciously sought compensation for failure and frustration in other spheres of life. We may even suspect that sexual life for some men does not really satisfy the inner urge of a natural appetite, but is simply a means of feeding their ego, not infrequently a matter of masculine pride.

Whatever the motive behind it, sex is an integral part of the scheme of life for every normal individual. If the patient is told that he should curtail his sex activity to a significant degree, he will likely become an emotional and mental invalid.

Sexual activities should not be resumed for at least six weeks to two months after a heart attack, and in special cases for as long as six months and occasionally even longer. If the patient becomes somewhat short of breath and is too greatly exhausted after sexual intercourse, he should wait until he gains a little more strength. A few individuals experience actual anginal pain at each act. For such persons it is advisable to take a nitroglycerine pill a little while before. At any rate, too great excitement can be avoided in marriage.

Aside from the deep satisfaction it affords in the psychological sphere, a sex life as close as possible to the normal should be the aim of all who have got safely through the more exacting period of a heart attack. As a matter of fact, for some persons the question of sex while convalescing becomes even more important than when they will be able to go back to work. This is actually a good sign, for it indicates that the patient is no longer in a panicky fear of death. Furthermore, it shows that he has regained a zest for life. Nothing will give a cardiac greater assurance than the knowledge that he will be able to lead a normal life, including, of course, sex.

10

Cholesterol and Calories

So MUCH has been written about cholesterol that the word to-day is a familiar one to practically everyone. During the past few years numerous articles have appeared in the press stating that scientists have found an exact correlation between fat in the national diet and the incidence of coronary heart disease. According to these studies, nations whose daily consumption of fat is low have a low incidence of coronary heart disease, while peoples whose fat consumption is particularly high have an extraordinarily high mortality rate from coronary heart disease.

The American diet, according to these studies, has the high-est content of fat. Also, Americans have the greatest incidence of heart attack of all nationalities. It has even been calculated that a Minnesota fireman has ten times as great a chance of suffering a heart attack as a Japanese fisherman, presumably because his fat consumption is so much greater than that of the Japanese.

Chances are you have never before heard of the Bantu in South Africa. Today, however, the Bantu have achieved ce-lebrity of a sort. It is said that the Bantu diet is extremely low in fat and coronary heart disease among them is almost a rarity. We should modify our diet accordingly.

Can You Eat Your Heart Out?

It would seem that we are eating ourselves into a heart attack. Those who became overly alarmed by such a prospect urge that we change our diet radically and cut down drastically on fats, especially those rich in cholesterol. It was not so long ago that people were warned to avoid eggs altogether, or at least limit them, since egg yolk is particularly rich in cholesterol.

Many scientists, however, question whether a possible connection between dietary fat and coronary heart disease can be established from population statistics alone. When the original studies were extended to more countries, it became evident that the mortality rate from heart attack does not always parallel the consumption of fat. To quote only one example: Fat consumption is very high in both Denmark and New Zealand. Yet the mortality rate from coronary heart disease is much higher in New Zealand than it is in Denmark.

Such a contradiction exists even among various countries in northern Europe. After examining the record of twenty nations in regard to fat and heart attack, Dr. Herman E. Hilleboe, New York State Commissioner of Health, and Dr. Jacob Jerushalmy, Professor of Bio-statistics at the University of California, found no relationship between fat consumption and mortality rates. However, this does not mean that fat and cholesterol have nothing to do with coronary heart disease.

Long before these popular articles made people cholesterol-conscious, an extraordinary amount of research had been carried out, to determine the possible role of diet in the development of coronary heart disease. Experimental work on animals, laboratory work, accurate measurements, and clinical observations brought out an enormous number of facts. Each new fact led to new questions, even more difficult to answer.

So it is that the question of fat in general and cholesterol in particular is far from being completely solved. Nevertheless, there is sufficient evidence to suggest that nutrition may be an important factor in bringing on deterioration of the coronary artery. Just exactly what the nutritional factor or factors are, and how they operate, no one pretends to know exactly. The greatest experts in the field differ widely in their conclusions.

You are not expected to be an arbiter in this scientific controversy. However, you should know something of the basic facts about which most scientists agree.

What Cholesterol Is

Deposits in the lining of the coronary artery consist largely of cholesterol. How does cholesterol get there?

Cholesterol is not some kind of poison, or an abnormal product of the body. Actually, cholesterol is perfectly normal and is an indispensable constituent of the body. It is present in many cells and in large quantities in the bile, where it helps digestion. It performs many other useful functions.

Some of the cholesterol is in the cells and some is carried in blood. Part of this cholesterol comes from the food we ingest and part of it is manufactured in the body itself, also from substances other than fat. Some persons have more cholesterol in the blood than others. The most natural supposition is that, in persons whose blood is too rich in cholesterol, the excess sticks to the lining of the arteries, among them the coronary itself. Tempting as this solution seems, extensive research does not bear it out.

The exact amount of cholesterol in the blood can easily be determined. Investigators found that many persons have an excessive amount of cholesterol in their blood, yet do not have the slightest trouble with their coronary. On the other hand, there are a great many people who have suffered a heart attack, yet the cholesterol content is normal, or maybe even below the average.

It is certain that there must be some other factor that determines whether the cholesterol that constantly bathes the walls of the arteries will be separated from the blood stream and stick to the wall of the artery.

A further complicating factor is that the degree of concentration of cholesterol in your blood does not depend on how much cholesterol you take in with your food. You may eat food very rich in cholesterol, yet in a short time your blood will have no greater concentration than it had before. On the other hand, you may stick to comparatively low cholesterol foods, yet your cholesterol content may remain the same.

Where Cholesterol Comes From

This is partly due to the fact that the body is capable of building up cholesterol from other substances than food. Only about half of the cholesterol in the body comes from food; the other half comes from the production of it in the body.

Some people inherit a constitution that can handle even large amounts of cholesterol in the blood without the slightest effect on the blood vessels. There are reports of several families in which the majority of the members, young and old, have high cholesterol levels, yet they are no more prone to coronary disease than others. On the other hand, there are individuals who cannot handle efficiently even small amounts of cholesterol.

Even though diet may play a role in the development of coronary heart disease, it certainly is not the only one. Other factors, such as heredity, active or sedentary life, emotions, the nature of the blood vessels, and many others, are involved in it.

But although diet is only one of the factors, it probably is one of them. Completely to disregard diet on the grounds that we do not know exactly what its role is would be just as serious a fallacy as the many fads, based on insufficient and often one-sided evidence, that have mushroomed into popularity.

To complicate matters still further, not all kinds of fats have the same effect on the cholesterol content of the blood. One kind of fat has a tendency to increase the cholesterol in the blood, while another kind actually causes it to be reduced.

First, it was thought that animal fats increase the cholesterol content of the blood, while those of vegetable origin either do not raise it or actually lower it.

Then some investigators discovered that such a distinction does not altogether hold true. In one study, the cholesterol content of the blood was measured in three groups of persons. The first group consisted of persons who followed an ordinary diet, including meat products. The second were so-called lacto-ovo-vegetarians; that is, they consumed such animal products as milk and eggs but eschewed meat in any form. The third group were "pure" vegetarians, persons who would not eat anything in any form from the animal kingdom. The investigators found the cholesterol content highest among non-vegetarians, considerably lower among lacto-ovo-vegetarians, and lowest of all among "pure" vegetarians, despite the fact that the latter group had practically the same proportion of fat in their diet as the non-vegetarians.

Studies were carried out among ethnic groups closely corresponding to these three groups—Peruvian Indians, Navaho Indians, American Trappist monks, and Cleveland Americans. Cholesterol levels were lowest among Peruvian Indians, largely "pure" vegetarians; somewhat higher among the Trappist monks, who consume egg and milk products; and highest of all among Americans.

The third kind of evidence that made distinction between animal and vegetable fats untenable was furnished by the example of the Eskimos. The Eskimos live on a high meat and high fat diet almost exclusively. The fat is derived from seal, walrus, or fish in general—again an animal source. Yet the average blood cholesterol content of Eskimos is considerably lower than that of the Canadians.

Chemical analysis shows that all fats contain two different kinds of fatty acids. One type is called a *saturated* fatty acid, the other *unsaturated*. *Saturated fats* raise the blood cholesterol level. *Unsaturated fats* either do not raise it or actually lower it.

You need not be a chemist to tell which kind of fatty acid is in the food you consume. In general, fat that is solid is a saturated fat, while one that remains liquid at room temperature is an unsaturated fat. As a rule, animal fat contains saturated fatty acids, while vegetable fats contain unsaturated fatty acids.

This is why, for example, "pure" vegetarians, who obtain the fat in their diet from vegetable source, have a low cholesterol level. But the thing is even more complicated. Margarine is of vegetable origin and, consequently, is high in unsaturated fatty acids. However, manufacturers add a substance that transforms it into saturated fat.

On the other hand, not all animal fat is saturated. Fat derived from fish, despite being of animal origin, contains unsaturated fatty acids. This explains why Eskimos have such low level of cholesterol in the blood.

Fats and Calories

Some investigators believe that the proportion of calories derived from fat to the total calories in the daily diet is more important than the amount of fat the person consumes. These investigators claim that if the proportion of fat is too high the cholesterol content of the blood will increase.

Consequently, they advocate cutting down on fat, but certainly not cutting it out altogether. Animal experiments have shown that too drastic a reduction of fat may actually be harmful. Rats whose daily diet was altered so that fats supplied less than 10 per cent of the total calories showed evidence of rapid aging. Fatty acids are needed for the absorption of various vitamins. The minimal basic requirement for human beings has never been established. Nevertheless, there is some evidence to indicate that fat is indispensable for health.

Dr. Irvine H. Page drastically reduced all fats in his own diet. Soon he began to suffer from intestinal disturbances, became markedly depressed and unduly irritable. Other doctors report weakness, stomach trouble, constriction of the chest, and sense of impending collapse in some patients on extremely low fat diets. Still others found no ill effects from the so-called rice diet, which is practically fat free.

These results are certainly contradictory. *But all these data relate largely to healthy people.*

For those who have suffered a heart attack low fat diet is probably important since, perhaps from an inborn deficiency of the system, some cannot handle cholesterol efficiently. Reduction of fat can be accomplished in part by trimming fat from meat, use of lean meats, and smaller servings. These persons should eat more fish, and less butter, margarine, whole milk, cheese (except cottage), bacon, and egg yolks.

A study now in progress at the Yale University Medical School casts further doubt about the value of low fat diets without taking into consideration other factors. Preliminary findings of Dr. Margaret M. Albrink indicate that a diet too low in fats and too high in carbohydrates might possibly raise the concentration in the blood of triglycerides, an important constituent of all kinds of fats. If these initial findings are confirmed by further study, the diet of some patients might have to be modified, but certainly not to any great extent.

But a comparatively low fat diet is not sufficient. Exercise can reduce the cholesterol level of the blood. Furthermore, by properly spacing fat intake a lower cholesterol level can be maintained.

There is still another reason why fat in the diet should be reduced. Some investigators proved by actual measurements that after a meal containing fat the blood tends to clot much more easily. This effect lasts for about an hour and a half after the meal. After a meal containing little or practically no fat, for the next six hours the tendency of the blood to clot will be even less than it was before the meal.

You will readily appreciate what this means when you remember that a greater tendency of the blood to clot may lead to thrombus formation in persons whose coronary artery is considerably narrowed. It must be stated, however, that other investigators were unable to confirm these findings.

One thing, however, seems certain, namely, that individuals differ markedly in their dietary requirements. Whether a person needs a certain type of diet depends on so many factors that *a diet list should come only from your doctor.*

Even though the entire question is far from being resolved, and although the greatest experts recognize that no absolute answer can be given with the present-day medical knowledge, you should certainly not succumb to any dietary fads recommended by non-experts. As the nutritional authorities of the Harvard School of Public Health, who reviewed the entire scientific evidence on nutritional factors in heart attack, have stated: "Although the statement 'a screwball needs a screwball diet' is facetious, it contains a germ of truth, and, we might add, such diets are usually recommended by 'screwballs.'"

Facts About the American Diet

From hearing and reading so much about heart attack today, many people believe that the incidence of heart attack has increased tremendously during the past few years, and that those living today are far more likely to suffer a heart attack than were their fathers and grandfathers. Indeed, heart specialists who have practiced for two or three decades report that they see more heart patients today than they saw when they started practicing. They, too, believe that the incidence has risen somewhat, but certainly not to such a frightening extent as most people think.

Just how great the increase is, no one knows exactly. For one thing, a far greater proportion of people now reach the age when coronary disease is likely to develop. For another, as all physicians recognize, diagnostic methods are far more accurate today than they were only two decades ago, so that many more cases are diagnosed correctly today. The increase may be partly due to these two factors.

What are the actual facts about the claimed increase in consumption of fat among Americans? No doubt you have read a good deal about the high fat content of the average American diet today. It is also said that we eat too much of the wrong kinds of fat with a corresponding decrease in consumption of unsaturated fatty acids that would tend to reduce the cholesterol content of the blood. How much truth is in such statements?

The amount of food available for the general population for each year is given in the records of the Agricultural Department dating back to 1910. From these records it might appear that Americans of this generation eat more fat than they did a generation ago. However, scientists who reviewed these data point out that from the available food at any period it cannot be estimated accurately how much of the food actually goes on the table.

A good deal of fat is discarded after the cooking of meats, bacon or fat fryings. This waste is much greater during periods of prosperity. How much fat is actually wasted and discarded can easily be judged from the tremendous collection of fat from kitchen waste during the war years. Furthermore, broiling is much more popular today than it was a generation or so ago. Consequently, less fat is used in the cooking of meat than formerly.

But there is a better way to judge food consumption today and in the past. A dietary survey of college men in a boarding club in 1891 showed that 44 per cent of the calories came from fat. A survey of the diet of women eating at college clubs in 1894 reported that 36 per cent of the calories came from fat. Even the Harvard Crew in 1898 consumed a diet providing 39 per cent of the total calories as fat.

Now, a study made in 1953 of adult women showed that on the average the customary diet contained from 36 to 46 per cent fat. So it is obvious that the American diet has not changed to any great extent during the past two generations.

We can give an even more striking illustration that eating habits have not greatly changed by comparing the Army rations in the past with those of today. A study of Army rations in western outposts in the late 1880's showed fat content almost identical with current U.S. Army rations. Even the proportion between animal and vegetable fats has not changed to any appreciable degree.

The reason many people think Americans today eat more fat than they used to is that they have been made more conscious of it because of the many popular articles on the subject.

All this leads to the conclusion that the average person need not worry about his customary diet, provided he is in good health. Any well-balanced diet will supply enough essential nutrients and adequate amounts of vitamins.

The American Heart Association appointed a special committee of five of the greatest experts in the field of nutrition to answer exactly this question. After reviewing all the scientific evidence, not a little of it developed by the scientists themselves from their previous work, and weighing all the pros and cons, the experts concluded that "the evidence at present does not convey any specific implications for drastic dietary changes, specifically in the quantity or type of fat in the diet of the general population, on the premise that such changes will definitely lessen the incidence of coronary or cerebral artery disease."

Diet and Heart Attack

The situation is far different for the person who has suffered a heart attack. For such a person the question is not whether his coronary has accumulated too much cholesterol deposit from too much fat in the past, but whether continued fat consumption may be harmful for him.

More and more evidence shows that low cholesterol diet, with special attention to the kind of fat in the diet, has proven beneficial to many patients.

Other investigators, however, have attributed the beneficial effect of such diet not to low cholesterol itself but to the fact that such diet is an excellent reducing diet. For overweight naturally places an extra burden on the heart. Overweight also tends to interfere with physical activity. For these reasons, reducing is highly important. With reduction in weight the blood cholesterol level usually falls.

Whatever the reason behind it, dietary regulation has proved to be probably the most important advance in treating coronary heart disease—as important, and perhaps even more so, as the use of anticoagulants.

Diet is particularly important for those who are overweight, for those whose cholesterol level is consistently high, and for persons who have a bad family history of early death of close relatives from heart disease. What kind of diet each person should follow if he is in any of these categories, only a physician can determine.

Naturally, no physician can give a detailed lecture to each patient. For those who are particularly interested in the whole subject of diet in coronary heart disease, there are several excellent books available at inexpensive prices.[1]

Some kinds of quack diet formulas are advocated by persons who lack scientific background in nutrition. Such fads may do no harm to the average person who has no urgent medical reason to follow a strict and accurate diet, and who wants to use it only for reducing. The worst thing that can happen to a healthy person who falls for any of these miracle diets is that he will not lose at all. At any rate, there are extremely few individuals who persist long enough to derive any benefit from these reducing fads, even if they happen to be fairly reasonable.

But for the person who has had a heart attack to tinker with such very often nonsensical diet fads is another matter. For this reason, *before you decide to follow any kind of diet, make sure who originates it.* It is not necessary that he have an imposing array of college degrees, but he should have an accurate knowledge of nutritional principles.

[1] Evelyn S. Stead and Gloria K. Warren, *Low Fat Cookery* (New York: McGraw-Hill, 1956). How to modify your favorite recipes.

Lester Morrison, M.D., *The Low Fat Way to Health and Longer Life* (Englewood Cliffs, N.J.: Prentice-Hall, Inc., 1958). The best and most practical for the average person with the average pocketbook, allowing enough variety in the menus and also containing useful suggestions how to shop for low fat foods. Sufficient information about fat content of all kinds of food.

11

Back to Work

THE GREATEST difficulty the average person has in trying to adjust his life under new conditions is that he does not know what he can do and what he should avoid. What a person can do without harming his heart depends largely on his cardiac reserve. By cardiac reserve is meant the ability of the heart to meet extra demands imposed on it by stress, either physical or mental.

Many persons regain virtually a normal cardiac reserve, and there is no reason whatever why they should not lead a perfectly normal life, provided, of course, that they do not dissipate their capacity in mental, emotional, or physical excesses.

By economizing with their resources and by setting up, so to say, a budget of activities, persons can lead a highly satisfactory and productive life. There are very few who cannot resume their former occupation, often without any restriction or with only a few not too severe ones. "It is a rare patient indeed who is fit for nothing."

How Heart Reserve Can Be Determined

During the last war there was an acute shortage of manpower in industry. In looking for a new source of labor, the War Manpower Commission turned its attention to those who were out of work because of some kind of physical handicap or because they had heart disease. Physicians who examined these people found that the vast majority of them could work. The judgment of the physicians was fully justified when these men proved themselves as productive and efficient as other workers in practically every job.

Following this happy experience, many of the largest industries set up a program of physical rehabilitation. During this program, physicians gradually evolved highly efficient methods by which the physical fitness of the prospective employee could be accurately evaluated. This evaluation is equally applicable to any kind of occupation—desk, executive or professional, as well as industrial. You are no longer left to guesswork to know how much you can do and what to avoid, and, what is equally important, how you should modify some aspects of your life so as to live a normal life within your individual capacity.

In evaluating a person's ability to take up a particular occupation, the physician considers, in general, two things. The first is how that person responds to various ordinary activities. The second is the accurate measurement of the function of the heart when the patient is subjected to various kinds of stresses.

How You Can Judge Your Fitness

One way you can tell whether you have been overdoing is how easily you tire after physical exertion. Being tired is not always a sign that you have overtaxed your heart. Fatigue is far more often the result of anxiety, emotional disturbance, or worry than of hard physical work.

Before you blame your heart, you should carefully observe what has brought on fatigue and, what is even more important, how long it lasts. If you still feel tired after a short rest, you can be almost certain it was due to anxiety, worry, or "nerves," and not to overexertion. If fatigue is due to overtaxing the heart, the tiredness disappears after a short rest.

Another way you can estimate the capacity of your heart

is to note when and under what conditions you become markedly short of breath. Excitement, a heavy meal, exposure to extremes of temperature, even a slight cold, may be accompanied by shortness of breath without indicating overburdening of the heart.

Even if excessive fatigue or shortness of breath is due to limitation of heart reserve, you can rearrange your life so as to conserve your resources by eliminating unnecessary details and, in general, by observing strict economy of energy expenditure. You will, perhaps, need more rest during the day or you may have to do things at a more leisurely pace, or take vacations from time to time.

In evaluating capacity and physical fitness, the physician will rely greatly on what the patient tells him about his own symptoms. He will first ask him how far he can walk on level ground and uphill, how many steps he can climb, and to what extent he can engage in ordinary home activities, without discomfort. Ability to engage in sexual activity without cardiac pain is an excellent gauge of heart reserve. Women patients are asked about their response to usual household chores, shopping, or carrying packages.

But the most important way the physician evaluates physical fitness is how well the patient can carry out various activities of the particular job he is engaged in.

A man who has been doing the same kind of work, whether physical or mental, for a good many years has learned to do his work in the most economical way. He does not fritter away his physical and mental energy on superfluous details. One of the secrets of why a trained athlete seems to perform so effortlessly is that he has eliminated all unnecessary motion.

For this reason, a middle-aged man will usually be better off if he returns to the job he had before rather than attempting to learn a new one. Just remember that when you do return to your old job you will be likely to tire more easily for the simple reason that you have been out of training for some time. This difficulty will disappear when you have become better conditioned.

Tests for Heart Capacity

The second way the physician can judge the capacity of the heart is by applying various tests by which he can measure accurately the function of the heart itself. In these tests, the patient is subjected to various standardized stresses. His response to them is measured by changes in blood pressure, output of the heart, breathing, electrocardiogram, oxygen consumption, and many others. From the magnitude of these changes, the physician has a good idea how well the person will stand up under stress. Exercise is one of the most commonly used stresses.

The simplest of these exercise tests is recording the patient's reaction to knee bending and to hopping. First, the physician counts the pulse rate and the rate of respiration, and measures the blood pressure. The patient is then asked to bend his knees twenty times. At the end of this exercise, in a healthy individual the pulse increases no more than 20 per minute, the blood pressure rises only slightly, and respiration is not speeded up appreciably. But the most important gauge of the person's heart reserve is how soon all these measurements return to normal. The pulse rate should return to normal two minutes after exercise. If it takes longer than that, it is an indication that the heart reserve is not quite up to par.

After the person has rested for a while, he is asked to hop 50 times on one foot. The pulse rate should not increase more than 30 per minute. In this test also, all measurements should return to normal within two minutes.

The Master Two-Step Test

Dr. Arthur M. Master devised an even more standardized exercise test. This test, which is the one most widely used by physicians, is called the Master two-step test. The apparatus for it consists only of two wooden steps, each nine inches high, joined together and facing both ways. The patient is asked to walk up these two steps, step down, and, turning around, walk over them again in the opposite direction. He has to make these trips for exactly one and a half minutes.

So that the results could be compared, Dr. Master prepared an accurate table showing how many trips a person has to make in a minute and a half, according to his age, sex, and weight. Naturally, a young man making the same number of trips does not place the same burden on his heart as an older one. In order to give you some idea how great the difference may be, a boy or girl from five to nine years old has to make 35 trips over the steps. A fifty-year-old man weighing 150 pounds must complete 20 trips, but only 17 if he weighs over 200 pounds. Incidentally, this again demonstrates the decided disadvantage of overweight. The man weighing 200 pounds expends as much energy in 17 trips as the man weighing only 150 pounds uses up in 20 trips.

This standardization according to age, weight, and sex makes it possible to compare the performance of each individual. After carrying out the exercise for the prescribed length of time, the effect of the two-step test on the patient's heart reserve is determined on the same principle as in the knee bending and the hopping tests. In addition to blood pressure, rate of breathing, pulse rate, and changes in electrocardiogram are also measured.

Naturally, immediately after the two-step test the heart will beat a little faster and the blood pressure will rise moderately. In healthy persons, both the pulse rate and the blood pressure should return to normal in no more than two minutes. In those whose heart reserve has been impaired, it takes much longer for both blood pressure and pulse rate to return to normal. Now, from the time required for these rates to return to normal, a score is made for each individual, and his heart reserve is judged by this score.

A far more accurate method of gauging the effect of the two-step test is to take an electrocardiogram both before and after the test. The electrocardiogram does not change, or changes only to a very slight degree, in subjects whose heart is normal. However, if the heart is not quite up to par, there will be definite changes in the pattern of the electrocardiogram. In this way the physician can discover impairment of the heart that otherwise would not have been evident.

The test is so simple that you may be tempted to try it out yourself on the steps at home and see how soon your pulse returns to normal. But you should not do this, especially if you have had a heart attack previously or suspect that your heart is not quite up to par. Simple as it may seem, the Master two-step test places considerable burden on the heart.

It is true that the test lasts only a minute and a half. However, this sudden and sharp increase may be too much for a heart not accustomed to such sudden changes and may actually damage it. The doctor will not allow a patient to perform the test if, in his judgment, he cannot do it safely.

On the Job

A few years ago Dr. R. C. Garry and his co-workers made an extensive study of the amount of work performed by clerks in a mine at Fife, Scotland. Using the calories burned up as a yardstick, they found that during the entire period of work these clerks averaged 1.7 calories per minute.

The investigators then continued the same measurements while the clerks were at home, engaged in usual home activities, in recreation, and in general what they customarily did away from the job. At the end of eight non-working hours they added up the calories used, and found that the energy expenditure averaged almost exactly three calories per minute. The mine clerks *"worked" nearly twice as hard at home as on the job.*

The case of the mine clerks was not an exceptional one. Sitting at a desk practically all the time during working hours and doing only mental work requires very little physical exertion. However, similar studies carried out in a wide range of other occupations, including factory workers, brought out that a great many, perhaps the majority, of occupations in America today require a surprisingly small amount of physical effort.

Data obtained on German workers in heavy industries revealed that an average expenditure of five calories per minute during the entire period of work does not cause undue fatigue and can be maintained without in any way overstepping human endurance. But the great majority of modern industrial jobs require an average energy expenditure of only half that much, or even less than that. This applies to desk work, professions, employment in stores—as a matter of fact, to any non-factory job, where the energy expenditure is even less than it is in the factory.

The average person after complete recovery from a heart attack, even though he feels in perfect health while still at home, is usually a bit apprehensive about the prospect of going back to work. He is afraid that the job will impose too much burden on his heart, and that maybe he will be unable to stand up to the effort required. Even after he has gone back, he is likely to be overcautious lest he overtax his heart. Yet the experience of all industrial physicians who have made follow-up studies of cardiacs employed in a great variety of factory work is that the *condition of 70 to 75 per cent of such workers actually improved while working,* or at least remained unchanged.

You *Should* Work

In the first place, as Dr. Paul Dudley White expressed it: "Work has a beneficial effect on body, mind, and soul in any occupation in which it is possible for the cardiac patient to engage. Idleness breeds unhappiness and is actually bad for the health."

In the second place, most heart attack victims regain virtually normal cardiac reserve. Normal cardiac capacity being so great, and energy requirements of practically all occupations nowadays being extremely low, *there is no danger whatever of overtaxing the heart.*

Working conditions have changed tremendously today. With all the modern labor saving devices, a good deal of physical effort has been eliminated. A generation or so ago factory work meant heavy and often exhausting labor. Today when machines do all the heavy work, a factory worker has it comparatively easy. As a rule, very little physical exertion is necessary. The stress involved in going back and forth from the job, the irritation involved in traffic conditions, may far exceed the actual energy the average worker expends at the job. Such labor saving applies with as much force to working conditions at the office or store. Perhaps we have become too soft, lead too sedentary a life, which is far more harmful for the heart than any possible damage from working too hard.

You can gain a more realistic view of the work involved in any occupation if you compare the expenditure required at the job with the expenditure involved in ordinary home activities. Dr. Robert A. Bruce of Seattle prepared a chart that compares energy expenditures of all kinds of occupations with that expended at home. He used as the basis of comparison the energy expended by the body at complete rest. He then calculated how much more energy is expended in various activities, at home, in industry, and on the farm.

From this chart you will see, for example, that a person walking upgrade expends about four times as much energy as when he is lying flat. But a bench worker expends only twice as much as compared with the resting condition.

Take a little closer look at these figures. While you are standing and talking you are expending very little more energy than while doing desk work. Notice also that the heaviest kind of industrial work will take out of you even less than walking fast on level ground. Of course, you may object that if you walked for eight hours it would make you awfully tired, and the chances are you would not be able to do it at all. And so you think you would not be able to do industrial work for eight hours either, even if it requires less exertion. But remember that nobody works steadily for the entire shift without a stop. There are plenty of intervals when the task is much easier. The expenditure is spread out over the entire working period.

This point will be more evident if you look at the chart, "On the Farm." Here you can see that the various tasks during the working day of a farmer vary enormously in terms of energy expenditure. You can see that carrying 100 pounds

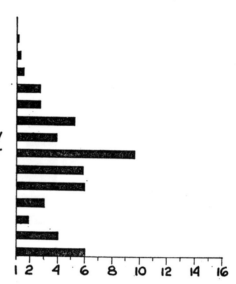

Figure 7a. ENERGY EXPENDITURE IN DAILY LIFE. (From Robert A. Bruce, M.D., "Evaluation of Functional Capacity in Patients with Cardiovascular Disease," *Geriatrics,* Vol. 12, No. 5, May, 1957)

upstairs requires 16 times the expenditure of the resting state, but that harrowing implies only about twice the expenditure while at rest. Naturally, farm work, like any other work, is never of a steady pattern. The task is rather exacting for a short time; then after a little rest comes some task that is rather easy. How all this adds up you can see from the chart, "In Industry," which lists the average daily expenditure of a hand farmer as less than four times as great as the resting state.

Meeting the Job's Requirements

The real question is: How well can the cardiac patient stand up even to these moderate requirements? We can give an accurate answer to this question.

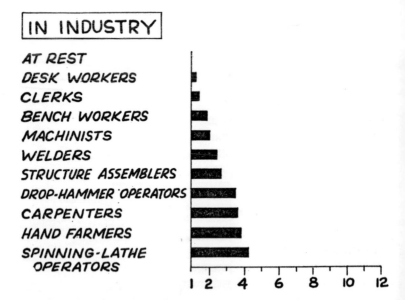

Figure 7b. ENERGY EXPENDITURE IN INDUSTRY. (From Robert A. Bruce, M.D., "Evaluation of Functional Capacity in Patients with Cardiovascular Disease," *Geriatrics,* Vol. 12, No. 5, May, 1957)

About two years ago, Drs. Amasa B. Ford and Herman K. Hellerstein, of Western Reserve University, Cleveland, Ohio, undertook a study that should be of particular interest to everyone who is contemplating going back to work after a heart attack, and equally so for persons who are already back at their former occupation. It was made in the factory itself, during a typical working day, so that it in no way resembled experimental conditions.

Drs. Ford and Hellerstein selected 36 employees of three large Cleveland manufacturing firms who had various kinds of heart disease, most of them persons who had recovered from a heart attack. All but one were men, ranging in age from twenty-four to seventy. They were workers in every major department of these three plants, which manufacture medium

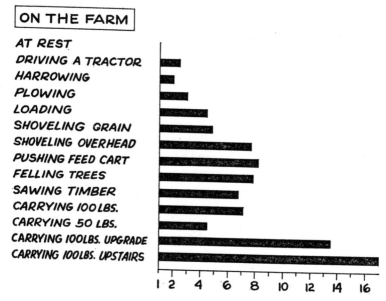

ON THE FARM

AT REST
DRIVING A TRACTOR
HARROWING
PLOWING
LOADING
SHOVELING GRAIN
SHOVELING OVERHEAD
PUSHING FEED CART
FELLING TREES
SAWING TIMBER
CARRYING 100 LBS.
CARRYING 50 LBS.
CARRYING 100 LBS. UPGRADE
CARRYING 100 LBS. UPSTAIRS

Figure 7c. ENERGY EXPENDITURE ON THE FARM. (From Robert
A. Bruce, M.D., "Evaluation of Functional Capacity in Patients
with Cardiovascular Disease," *Geriatrics,* Vol. 12, No. 5, May,
1957)

and light metal products, and are representative of the type of
industry employing one-third of the working population of
Cleveland and vicinity.

They were bench workers, foremen, machine operators,
maintenance workers, warehousemen, and included planning
clerks, millwrights, inspectors, supervisors, plant guards—in
short, persons performing jobs requiring different degrees of
skill and varied amounts of energy expenditure. Thus, the
jobs ranged from menial to managerial and from sedentary to
active. Consequently, the findings can be applied to most other
occupations and professions, insofar at least as the actual
work involved is concerned.

In order to compare ability, efficiency, and effect of the
work of these cardiacs at the job, the investigators selected 26

normal employees, matched as nearly as possible with the cardiacs as to age, occupation, and skill, who constituted the control group.

All the subjects, cardiacs and healthy employees, reported at the company dispensary fifteen minutes before the shift. After the purpose and method of the study was explained to them, they were equipped with a number of special apparatuses to measure their exact energy expenditure, and also the effect of the work on their heart. During the working day, a number of different measurements were made, so that every phase of work was covered. These measurements in no way interfered with their usual work.

From the data thus amassed, Drs. Ford and Hellerstein were able to gain a complete picture of the load imposed on the heart throughout the day and the ability of the cardiacs to meet the various requirements. After the study was over, these doctors collected all the data, analyzed them, and then were able to announce their conclusions.

From these very extensive data, we select those that are particularly pertinent in answering the two main questions. First, how the effort required by the cardiacs for a given task compared with that required by healthy workers. Second, and even more important, how well the heart stood up under actual working conditions. But before we can answer either of these questions, we need to find out how much energy the cardiacs used up in performing the various jobs, and what it amounted to for the entire shift.

During the 8½ hour shift, the entire group of cardiacs averaged slightly less than two calories per minute, that is, no more than about twice the energy needed during complete rest.

This, of course, included all types of work. As can be expected, one type of work required more effort, others less. Nevertheless, the range of energy expenditure for all types of work was very small. An electrician, for example, used up no more than 1.25 calories per minute. But the energy expenditure did not exceed three calories per minute in any kind of work.

It seems that the job of a janitor is one of the most exacting, and yet even his calorie expenditure was only slightly over 2.5 calories per minute. Only a stock piler worked hard enough to average around three calories per minute.

Naturally, as we have pointed out, no one works at exactly the same pace throughout the shift. Some part of the job may require greater effort, while at other times the worker will have an extremely light task. And this point is particularly important in the case of so-called cardiacs. A sudden strain may be more harmful than steady work at a somewhat higher level of energy expenditure. But even in jobs requiring more effort at times, for perhaps ten minutes or so, these workers seldom needed to expend more than four calories per minute at peak levels. The investigators found that the majority of the jobs followed a steady pattern of energy expenditure throughout the shift, and that the requirements of the heart hardly changed at all.

For supervisors and those engaged in maintenance work, walking made up the bulk of the energy demand. A pedometer was attached to each subject's belt, so that how much he walked during a shift could be accurately measured.

Twelve men in this kind of job walked more than five miles, and two, more than ten miles, on the job. Since the walking was at a slow pace, it required considerably less than three calories per minute. Even so, when the calorie expenditure of all activities, including walking, was added up for the entire shift, it averaged around 2.5 calories per minute.

This is an important point to remember if you are a professional man, insurance man, store-worker, and so forth, for in such occupations walking will require more energy expenditure than anything else you do.

Now, as to the first question: How did the energy expenditure of the cardiacs compare with that of healthy workers doing the same kind of work?

There was practically no difference in the energy expenditure of these two groups. In other words, the cardiacs did not have to work any harder to accomplish the same purpose. As Drs. Ford and Hellerstein stated:

> . . . there is no evidence in the present study that workers with compensated heart disease are compelled to make any greater demands upon their reserves in terms of pulse rate, pulmonary ventilation or oxygen utilization in order to perform this type of factory work than are their healthy co-workers.

As for the second question: Is work itself, and in this case industrial, which certainly is more exacting than other occupations, in any way harmful to the heart?

Electrocardiograms, blood pressure reading, and many other more complicated tests performed during the work at stated intervals definitely showed that there was at no time any change in the function of the heart. *The hearts of the cardiacs stood up exactly as well to the particular task as the hearts of the perfectly healthy workers.*

The fact is that the majority of occupations require no more effort than ordinary home activities, and frequently even less. No doubt it was this consideration that prompted Drs. Ford and Hellerstein to remark: "Little wonder that many cardiac patients prefer to work than to remain at home."

12

Angina Pectoris

AT THE July 21, 1768, meeting of the College of Physicians of London, Dr. William Heberden, a distinguished British physician, read a paper about a disorder of the breast previously unknown to the medical profession. With this masterpiece of accurate observation the history of the knowledge of coronary disease really begins. So penetrating and remarkable was Heberden's description that most of his little treatise could be reproduced without any changes in the most modern medical textbook of today. Because of "the seat of it, and sense of strangling and anxiety with which it is attended," he proposed to call this disorder *Angina Pectoris,* from the Latin words for "strangling" and "chest." And that is how it is known today.

> Those who are afflicted with it [he wrote] are seized, while they are walking, and more particularly when they walk soon after eating, with a painful and most disagreeable sensation in the breast, which seems as if it would take their life away, if it were to increase or to continue; the moment they stand still, all this uneasiness vanishes. In all other respects, the patients are, at the beginning of this disorder, perfectly well, and in particular have no shortness of breath, from which it is totally different.
>
> After it has continued some months, it will not cease so instantaneously upon standing still; and it will come by any disturbance of the mind. . . .
>
> When a fit of this sort comes on by walking, its duration is very short, as it goes off almost immediately upon stopping. . . .

. . . [It] most usually attacks only those who are above fifty years of age. . . .

The *os sterni* [breastbone] is usually pointed to as the seat of this malady, but it seems sometimes as if it was under the middle or upper part, but always inclining more to the left side and sometimes there is joined with it a pain about the middle of the left arm. . . .

. . . [Its nature] will readily present itself to any one, who considers the sudden manner of its coming on and going off; the long intervals of perfect ease; the relief afforded by wine and spirituous cordials; the influence, which passionate affections of the mind have over it. . . .

. . . [It is] a distemper hitherto so unnoticed, that it has not yet, as far as I know, found a place or a name in the history of diseases.

Although Dr. Heberden described the symptoms of angina pectoris with remarkable clarity, it is evident that he did not understand the true nature of the disease. Shortly after his treatise was published, Dr. Edward Jenner, who was later to introduce vaccination against smallpox, came to the conclusion from his autopsy work that angina pectoris was due to a diseased condition of the coronary artery. But Jenner's view was not generally accepted, and until comparatively recent times it was thought that angina pectoris had nothing to do with coronary heart disease. Today, as the result of accurate research work, we know that in about 90 per cent of cases the cause is coronary artery disease. In the other 10 per cent, angina is due to some other kind of heart disease, or to some other condition such as, for example, pernicious anemia. Here, however, we are concerned only with angina brought on by coronary artery disease.

What Causes Angina?

The anginal attack occurs when a tiny portion of the heart muscle is suddenly deprived of a sufficient amount of oxygen. Oxygen is carried to the heart muscle by the blood that flows through the branches of the coronary artery. How much oxygen the heart needs at the moment depends on how hard it has to work to supply a sufficient amount of blood to the various portions of the body. If you are at rest or asleep, demand for blood will be at a minimum. But if you are running, the muscles of the leg will need a good deal more blood, and so the heart has to pump that much more vigorously. The same happens if you are excited or upset, for now the brain telegraphs an urgent demand for more blood. In either case, all the branches of the coronary artery, even the smallest twigs on the arterial tree, expand evenly to allow more blood to flow through them. If for any reason one of these branches fails to keep pace with the rest, the tiny portion of the heart supplied by that particular branch will be deprived of a sufficient amount of oxygen. The result of this deprivation will be pain.

This is how anginal attack is brought on. This deprivation can occur only if that branch had been severely narrowed down by fatty deposits. Yet such narrowing of one or even many sections of the coronary artery does not necessarily lead to anginal attack. A person may have very extensive and widespread narrowing of a number of branches and yet never suffer anginal attack. On the other hand, there are some with minimal lesions of the coronary who suffer from frequent anginal pain. Severity of pain or frequency of anginal attacks does not necessarily indicate the extent of damage to the coronary artery.

What is the difference between angina and heart attack?

There is a difference, and an important one. In the case of heart attack, a portion of the heart muscle is deprived of blood usually because a blood clot shuts off the blood supply permanently, so that that portion of the heart muscle dies out. In the case of angina pectoris, the deprivation is only temporary, lasting for perhaps three to five minutes. The heart muscle is not damaged at all. After this extremely short period, the muscle again receives its due share of blood and is none the worse off for the episode.

Some angina sufferers experience numerous seizures, perhaps as many as twenty, practically every day, yet they live for many, many years.

A coronary artery that is narrowed down in one, two, or

even more places is still able to deliver all the blood needed for ordinary activities. If the demand for extra blood is slow and gradual, even if the coronaries are narrowed in many portions, there will be enough time for them to expand sufficiently for all the needed blood to be delivered to all parts of the heart muscle. However, if the demand is too sudden and too abrupt, the narrowed branch will not have enough time to respond properly. The pain that results from it usually forces the person to stop whatever he was doing. The demand for blood is thus decreased, and the balance of circulation is soon re-established.

The Anginal Attack

The attack is not actually a sharp pain but a sense of heaviness in the chest, a feeling of tightness, stretching, boring, aching, burning, or of a vise-like character.

The onset is seldom sudden, but the pain builds up gradually and gets worse as the attack progresses. To the sufferer himself it seems to last for a very long time. Actually, it lasts from two to five minutes, seldom longer. If the victim stops all activity immediately at the slightest indication that a seizure is coming on, no actual pain will develop, although he will have some slight soreness in the chest for half an hour or so afterward. It is highly characteristic of anginal attack that, unlike other kinds of pain, it promptly ceases when the person rests and remains absolutely quiet.

Some victims have learned by experience that the best thing to do is to stop immediately whatever they have been doing. Others, however, are too impatient and, knowing they will get over it anyhow, continue to work despite the discomfort.

This latter attitude is an entirely wrong one. The attack means that one tiny part of the heart does not receive enough blood, and as long as that condition exists the supply will not be restored. The heart can stand such deprivation for a short time. But if the condition is allowed to continue for an unnecessary length of time the heart may suffer some slight damage. Repeated deprivation of the heart muscle may eventually lead to permanent damage.

The other most characteristic feature of anginal attacks is that the pain usually radiates, that is, spreads, to other parts of the body, usually to the left arm, sometimes as far as the elbow, and less frequently to the wrist or fingers. Also characteristic is that the seizures follow a definite pattern in every individual as to how the pain spreads and under what particular conditions it comes on.

The frequency of the attacks varies greatly from individual to individual. Most patients have only occasional seizures weeks or even months apart. Others experience them almost regularly, and occasionally even more than once a day. However, by learning the particular kind of exertion that brings on attacks you can avoid most of them.

A twinge around your heart does not necessarily mean you have angina pectoris. There are many conditions that cause chest pain and that may be mistaken for angina. Sharp and sticking pain so frequent around the heart is more likely to be due to fatigue, anxiety, or nervous tension. The pain or ache in such cases may even spread to the shoulder or down the arm. But here is an important distinction. Such pain is felt on the side of the chest where the tip of the heart is, never under the breastbone as in true anginal seizure. Furthermore, it comes on after exertion or excitement, while true angina occurs during exertion or excitement. Besides, this kind of pain is not relieved by nitroglycerine, as it invariably is in the case of angina.

Leave it to your doctor to decide what the pain really means. Do not jump to the conclusion you have angina every time you have a pain in your chest.

Who Is Likely to Have Angina?

Angina pectoris is predominantly a disease of middle age and beyond. It is estimated that anywhere from 90 to 95 per cent of patients are past the age of forty when they experience the first seizure, but around 75 per cent are past fifty. Two investigators found that the average age of onset for men is fifty-six, and for women, fifty-eight. Men outnumber women at the ratio of from 3 to 1 to 6 to 1.

Occupations involving brain work and a good deal of responsibility are particularly prone to predispose to angina. Managers, executives, doctors, lawyers, are said to be particularly susceptible. Similarly, social status is said to play a definite role in it.

It is much more probable that in the last analysis heredity determines the likelihood of developing angina pectoris in later life. Angina is strikingly frequent among parents, brothers, or close relatives of the patient. There is also some evidence that certain constitutional characteristics may predispose the individual to it. Many of the victims are of the short and stocky type, short-necked and barrel-chested, most often overweight. We shall see later that it is precisely such individuals who, although not exclusively so, are also more prone to have a heart attack.

On the emotional side, many of the patients are aggressive, overambitious, inclined toward emotional excesses, quick-tempered, or overly sentimental, which tendencies they usually attempt to repress. Nevertheless, there are many individuals who, before they acquired the disease, were calm, quiet, easygoing, and in many respects the exact opposite of the above types. These, of course, will have little difficulty in properly adjusting to new conditions imposed by anginal attacks.

Those of an uneven temperament need to exercise a good deal of self-discipline to attain the more peaceful state of mind so important in reducing the frequency of the attacks. Several studies have shown that these desirable changes in general attitude pay off handsomely by reducing both the frequency of the attacks and the occasions that usually provoke them.

What You Can Expect

A number of years ago Drs. White, Bland, and Miskall published a follow-up study of 497 men and women with angina. The minimum period of observation for each of these patients covered twelve years, but in many cases considerably longer than that. The average duration of the ailment for 445 patients was almost exactly eight years. The other 52 were still alive on an average of 18.4 years after they first experienced an anginal attack. This, it should be repeated, is only the average, for quite a number have already lived for a considerably longer time than the average for the whole group.

If you take into consideration the fact that somewhat over 70 per cent of them were past fifty years of age when first stricken with the disease, you can see that for these persons angina pectoris did not appreciably shorten life expectancy, if at all. One physician reported the remarkable case of a woman who was alive 33 years after her first attack. In their report, these doctors pointed out the importance of strict observance of general rules for considerably prolonging life expectancy.

The majority of persons, including even those who suffer attacks frequently, are not at all handicapped by the disease. Some patients become altogether free of attacks for many months, and occasionally even for years. In others, anginal seizure may disappear completely, the patient being apparently cured.

What no doubt happens in such cases is that a satisfactory collateral circulation has been established, so that all parts of the heart receive enough oxygen even under conditions of stress. Even though the condition is likely to remain unchanged, how long you'll live after the first attack and how well you'll be able to adjust to the condition so that it will not interfere with your work, will depend a good deal on you. The most important thing is for you to do everything possible to avoid bringing on an attack.

Most people who experience an anginal seizure for the first time are frightened and expect to die with the next one. On the other hand, those who have had angina for many years and have found out that it is not dangerous, are likely to take little notice of it and neglect to take necessary precautions to avoid attacks. After all, they reason, a little pill of nitroglycerine gives prompt and complete relief, so why worry about it?

Yet both of these attitudes are wrong, and both may be harmful. The great anxiety that exaggerated fear is bound to provoke is certainly not good for the coronaries. On the other hand, long-continued neglect of the condition may lead to permanent damage to the heart. It is important to appraise the situation correctly and to be neither overly frightened nor too unconcerned.

But if, despite all precautions, you do have more or less frequent attacks, there are highly effective drugs that give complete relief.

Treatment

The best drug for angina pectoris is, unquestionably, nitroglycerine. Practically every patient carries in his pocket those indispensable little pills. Just one pill gives complete relief in one or, at most, two minutes.

Despite the fact that its efficiency and complete safety has been well established over many years, some persons still hesitate to take it regularly because of a possible unpleasant side-effect, such as fullness of the head, a throbbing sensation in the face, and occasionally slight dizziness. These unpleasant side-effects can almost invariably be avoided by reducing the size of the dose. Actually, a dose consisting of $\frac{1}{200}$ grain is just as effective as a dose twice as large.

Others are afraid to take nitroglycerine regularly for fear that it will be harmful in the long run. The fact is that repeated use is not harmful at all. There are patients who take as many as twenty or even more tablets in a day without the slightest harmful effect.

If you have not taken nitroglycerine before, your doctor will advise you to sit down or to support yourself when you take it for the first time, for it may cause dizziness. After you have found out your reaction to it and have become accustomed to it, you will be unlikely to experience dizziness. Doctors prescribe the drug in a form that will be absorbed very rapidly so that the effect will appear as quickly as possible. It is a good plan for you to crush the tablet and hold it under your tongue to assure rapid absorption.

Although nitroglycerine is cheap and safe to use, it is not necessary for a person to take it every time he has a mild attack. Stopping immediately the particular activity that threatens to bring on a full-scale attack will usually prevent it altogether. But if after a minute or so no relief is apparent, the patient should not hesitate to take a pill immediately. Nitroglycerine is very helpful not only in relieving an attack but also in preventing one from coming on. A person may have to perform, from time to time, more or less strenuous work that would ordinarily bring on an attack. However, if he takes a pill shortly before he intends to do something unusually strenuous he can prevent an attack. This allows the person to perform even somewhat heavy work without ill effect.

Just because nitroglycerine is effective in giving prompt relief and is perfectly harmless, it should never serve as an excuse for not taking proper precautions. Any kind of exertion that brings on an attack should be carefully avoided. There is no sense in causing oxygen deprivation for the heart, even for a short time, if it can be prevented.

Another drug that is highly effective and is even more prompt of action is amyl nitrite. It comes in pearl form. The drug is more expensive and, besides, has some drawbacks. It has a rather pungent odor, and it has to be crushed in a handkerchief, so that it is more troublesome to use.

Quite a number of different kinds of drugs have been developed either to prevent the occurrence of another attack or at least to reduce the frequency. These preparations aim at improving exercise tolerance by increasing coronary circulation. Some of these have been found effective for some patients, but not for all. The only way a physician can determine which drug will be effective is by giving each a trial. He may find just the one you need. At any rate, you must *leave it entirely to your doctor to prescribe the exact medication suitable for you.*

Besides any of these drugs, your doctor will probably prescribe some form of sedative drugs, the action of which is to allay anxiety and to circumvent too great an emotional upset, thus preventing situations likely to lead to an attack. Sleeping powders which assure a good night's rest sometimes are necessary for persons who are too tense to be able to procure a restful sleep.

Alcohol in small amounts has been found to be greatly helpful for patients with angina pectoris. Dr. Heberden, in the paper mentioned above, had already recognized the beneficial effect of "wine and spirituous cordials." It has been found out recently that alcohol does not dilate the coronary artery as was previously claimed. Its usefulness is due, rather, to the fact that it greatly reduces tensions of all kinds, calms the nerves, and contributes to a feeling of well-being. It is especially useful for older persons for its generally calming effect. Needless to say, overindulgence in any form of alcohol may have the exact opposite effect by encouraging the person to overactivity. However, one or two drinks at bedtime, or one or two glasses of wine with meals, are very helpful.

How to Avoid an Attack

Of all kinds of physical activity, walking is the one most likely to provoke an anginal attack. You may be able to walk on level ground without any ill effect. Yet if you walk the same distance up even the slightest incline you may bring on an attack. The pace also has a good deal to do with it. You may be able to walk a mile or even more slowly, without any discomfort. But if you walk more rapidly not more than half a block you may experience an attack. Consequently, everyone who is subject to angina should walk at what has been called a "banker's stride," and should frequently stop for a minute or so.

The Germans call angina sufferers "window shoppers," for they stop frequently and pretend to be looking at a shop window to avoid embarrassment. But in order to gain relief, it is not enough just to slow down the pace. The patient must stop altogether.

Curiously, some patients have an attack early in the morning but then, after a short period of rest, are able to perform more or less strenuous work for the rest of the day without suffering any ill effect at all. In other persons, exactly the same amount of extra work will usually provoke a fresh attack. Investigators, using a stair-climbing test, measured the exact amount of extra work that can be performed without pain. They found that each individual has his own schedule, above which he must not go. You can find out by your own experience what your limit is and, thus, avoid overexertion.

Food is another important precipitating factor. If you attempt even slight exertion shortly after a heavy meal, you are much more likely to experience a seizure than on an empty stomach. It is important, therefore, to rest after each meal. It is also advisable to eat lighter meals five times a day rather than three heavy ones. Cold is another precipitating factor, especially in windy weather. Cold decreases exercise tolerance. Cold bed sheets or even a cold drink may provoke an attack, and so may stepping into a cold bath. Nose and face seem especially susceptible. So if at all possible, you should avoid any exposure to cold. It is important that you wear warm clothing during the winter months, including gloves.

Emotions

Some patients regularly have an attack of angina in the morning after walking only a block or two to work. But the same person may walk the same distance on his way home without the slightest discomfort. Here the state of mind, worry or anxiety, and not the physical exertion, serves as a trigger mechanism in provoking an attack. It is easy to tell the victim of angina to avoid all possible sources of minor frictions at home or at work. But for him to put it into practice is another matter. Many angina sufferers are ambitious, hard-working, always on the go. For them radically to change a lifetime habit, and even more, a fundamental attitude, often presents an almost insurmountable obstacle.

When an overactive person suffers an anginal attack for the first time and learns about the true nature of his affliction, he may react to it in an unexpected way. He may become extremely pessimistic about his outlook, expecting to die any minute. On the other hand, especially if he is of an impatient make-up, he may decide to defy his fate and drive himself even more relentlessly.

Both such attitudes, the one of resignation and the defiant one, are equally harmful. Constant fear of imminent death can lead only to anxiety, worry, and heightened tension, all of which are highly conducive to a new attack. Such a patient needs, more than anything else, the kind of reassurance that only a complete knowledge of the real nature of his heart condition can give. Instead of brooding, he should learn that the probabilities are all in his favor. His chances for a long and useful life are always good. So far as his occupation is concerned, the chances are that he won't have to change it at all.

Nevertheless, he will have to change his habits somewhat and adjust himself to the situation. Such adjustments need not be major ones. An optimistic view, fully justified by facts, will help more than anything else to restore confidence and to attain a peaceful acceptance of possible limitations imposed by angina. Voluntary invalidism, often the result of exaggerated fear, will invariably lead to deterioration of the heart reserves because of self-imposed curtailment of all activities. But even more than lack of exercise, the resulting worry and fretfulness and an unavoidable sense of frustration, especially for a person who has been active all his life, actually impose a great burden on the heart. A vicious circle sets in.

Those who adopt a defiant attitude and try to work off an attack by even more vigorous exercise unnecessarily increase the momentary oxygen deprivation of the heart muscle by overstraining its ability to recover promptly from it. This tends to increase the frequency of the attacks, which, in turn, cannot fail to cause irritability, another trigger mechanism for further attacks.

Moderation in all matters, including matters both of mind and body, is the best preventative for considerably reducing the frequency of the attacks.

Rest and Exercise

Long hours of work without interruption, especially under constant tension, is the worst possible condition for anyone with angina, even though the attacks may be infrequent and rather mild.

First of all, you should never have to hurry to work in the morning, rushing to catch a bus or subway after a hurried breakfast. It will pay you to get up half an hour earlier so that you can have a leisurely breakfast and plenty of time to get to work.

If it can be arranged, you should take a short rest in the middle of the morning. For those who can manage it, a short nap in mid-afternoon will help refresh mind and body.

Never start any activity, no matter how light, for at least 45 minutes after the evening meal. It probably isn't even necessary to mention that you must not eat a heavy meal in the evening.

Early to bed should be the rule. If necessary, you should take a sleeping powder to assure an undisturbed night's sleep.

Although it is not always possible, it is advisable to take two vacations every year, one during extremely hot weather in the summer and another during severe cold in the winter. Besides avoiding undesirable extremes of temperature, the patient will benefit greatly from this restoration of physical and mental energy.

For those who have angina in a severe form with frequent attacks, occasional absolute bed rest for a few weeks can be extremely helpful. But prolonged stay in bed can have just the opposite effect if it leads to a pessimistic attitude and destruction of morale.

While it is true that a person subject to anginal attack should do everything in a leisurely manner and avoid anything that puts a sudden strain on his heart, he need not lead a completely sedentary life. On the contrary, mild exercises are very helpful and, if carried out sensibly, will actually build up a tolerance for physical exertion. Needless to say, exercise should never be continued until the person becomes exhausted. It should be increased gradually and cautiously.

If you can afford it, take a "cure" from time to time in some health resort, either in this country or in Europe. Here you will receive expert massage, special baths at prescribed times, supervised exercises, special diet, and follow a strictly regulated schedule. You will come back home greatly improved, with frequency of attacks greatly reduced and your work tolerance markedly increased. Actually, these health resorts or sanitariums for cardiacs have no secret formulas, and certainly mineral waters or baths have no specific curative values. The benefit is due entirely to the fact that you have got away from everyday worries in business and from domestic stress, live in beautiful and pleasant surroundings and, above all, follow a strict regimen under expert care.

For those of us who cannot afford such luxury, home treatment can be just as effective if we are willing to obey the rules. As a matter of fact, a "rest cure" carried out at home will be even more beneficial in many cases than an expensive course of treatment that you can ill afford. When you take your regular vacation, you can arrange a schedule that will include all the usual benefits of a health resort.

As for year-round recreation at home, of course you won't be able to take part in any strenuous sport. You'll be able to play golf, but be sure you have a caddy, and forget the score. Swimming should be avoided, not because it is too strenuous but because it may prove disastrous if you should have an attack away from the shore.

You may decide to retire completely if you have reached the usual age of retirement. In that case, be sure you have some other interest to take the place of your usual occupation. Retirement always presents serious problems, even for those who do not have a heart condition. Time lies heavily on the hands of the unfortunate person who has nothing to do and all the time in the world to do it in. Eventually he will become bored with his whole existence. Boredom and listlessness certainly are never conducive to peace of mind. Besides, such persons

inevitably become addicted to a sedentary life, since they have no incentive to do anything.

If you have an old hobby or interest, revive it. Or acquire a new one. Some of the "oldsters" who have taken up some hobby for which they never had enough time before are the happiest of individuals. Some of them, because they lend to their new interest the same zest and drive they formerly expended on their job, actually accomplish some really worthwhile goals in some other field.

You'll also have more time for recreation than you ever had before. You can go to the movies, watch your favorite TV program, play cards. But avoid seeing movies or TV programs that are overly exciting as they might bring on a fresh attack. And playing cards even for small amounts is hardly advisable as it may cause some chagrin.

Are You a Candidate
for Heart Attack?

13

Age and Sex

No DOUBT you have read a good many articles in the press that tell in a convincing manner what type of person is particularly prone to a heart attack. Some of these incriminate the terrific stress of modern life; the great responsibility that goes with an executive position; or too many cigarettes; but, most prominently, blame is placed on too much fat in the diet.

Other articles point out that a surprisingly large percentage of heart attack victims are of a certain body build; that is, the short, stocky, muscular, eminently masculine type. Most such articles are based on extensive research by scientists of the highest competence in their field, and are written in admirable manner. If they are misinterpreted by the general public, it is certainly no fault of the writers.

The average person reading such articles jumps to the wholly unwarranted conclusion that everyone who consumes too much fat, is under a constant stress of mental work, smokes too many cigarettes, or who is a short and stocky type, will invariably develop coronary heart disease. It is true that many cardiacs are of a certain body build. Many others come from a family heavily overladen with heart disease. The incidence of heart attack among doctors, for example, with their irregular hours and heavy responsibility, is the greatest among all occupations. Any of these factors, and many more, plays a role in rendering a person susceptible to heart attack. But none of these factors alone could possibly play a deciding role.

The Factor of Age

The overwhelming majority of persons who suffer a heart attack are between the ages of forty and seventy. Several studies put the percentage as somewhere between 83 and 90 per cent.

Hence it would appear at first glance that heart attack and its underlying cause, deterioration of the coronary artery, are the result of the wear and tear of years. As a matter of fact, until comparatively recent times physicians universally held that aging is some kind of disease in itself, the body being worn out by the relentless grindings of use and abuse.

Recent medical studies, however, have shown that this conception is not true at all. It is true that the skin of older persons becomes wrinkled because it dries out and loses its elasticity; the hair turns white because of the loss of pigment. However, the vital organs retain their vigor and functional capacity to an astonishing degree well up to advanced years.

Measurement at different age levels of the various hormonal substances manufactured daily by the body have demonstrated that, except for the male and the female hormones, the amount does not diminish to any great extent, at least not to such a degree as to interfere with the basic needs of the body. The individual red blood cells are being constantly worn out, but long before they lose their usefulness they are destroyed and in about three months are replaced with brand new blood cells. This is true throughout life. So in one respect, at least, a ninety-year-old man is as young as a twenty-year-old youth. Within obvious and specific limitations, the body can function adequately and creditably up to the end of the natural life span.

In the new conception of aging and old age, if a person gets old before his allotted time it is because something went wrong in some part of his system, and not because his tissues wore out by the corroding action of the years. This view removes the element of the unavoidable that would compel us to resign to the burden of old age as something inevitable.

In the past few years an entirely new branch of medicine, called gerontology, has arisen, which deals with the ailments of elderly persons. Gerontology attacks vigorously many of the problems of old age that until now had been regarded as beyond the power of medicine. The results are so gratifying that physicians are today far more optimistic about older persons and have succeeded in at least mitigating conditions that accompany aging.

If these general observations are correct for the entire body and its various organs, they are equally applicable to atherosclerosis of the coronary artery. Medical science has found that accumulation of fatty deposit occurs because something has gone wrong with the complex chemistry of the body, and not because of the advance of years. This revolutionary concept of atherosclerosis as the result of a number of physical and chemical changes in the body has radically altered the medical approach to the problem of coronary disease.

Coronary Disease Not the Toll of Age

As long as it was thought that coronary disease is the inescapable toll exacted by advancing years, no attempt was made to do anything about it. Now that it is known that a number of factors are involved in it, some of which are controllable and can be eliminated, the former pessimistic attitude has been abandoned. We know much better today how to arrange the life of those who have recovered from a heart attack in order to increase their life expectancy and to forestall, as much as possible, the occurrence of further heart attack.

What are the facts that led gradually to the conception of atherosclerosis as a definite disease process and not the result of aging?

First of all, there is the undeniable fact that heart attack is not confined to older persons. Although extremely rare, a number of undoubted instances of heart attack in babies and young children have been reported. Among men in their twenties and thirties, it is far more frequent than is generally realized. A number of soldiers in World War II came down with heart attack, and proportionately even more during the Korean War, not because conditions were more exacting during the Korean War but simply because by that time diagnostic methods were far more accurate, and many more cases were recognized. It is obvious that in young adults and in children age could not possibly have been the cause of changes in the coronary artery.

Again, quite a number of persons of advanced age have perfectly normal coronary arteries. Dr. Charles K. Friedberg, who examined at autopsy the hearts of a great many persons past the age of seventy who had died from some other causes, found that a surprisingly large percentage of these had coronaries remarkably free of any involvement.

Another strong evidence against the aging theory is that the incidence of heart attack does not rise exactly according to age. If severe deterioration of the coronary were due to age alone, you would expect that the older a person gets the more likely he would be to suffer a heart attack. Yet reliable statistics in this regard show that this is not the case.

This striking fact was brought out in an extremely interesting and, in many respects, unique study published recently by Dr. Louis Sigler. Dr. Sigler compiled an accurate history of 1,700 patients (1,302 males and 398 females) who had suffered a heart attack. Among the many facts observed, he recorded the age of occurrence of heart attack for each patient. The ages of occurrence ranged from twenty to ninety-three years. In order to eliminate the factor of sex, which we shall consider in the next section of this chapter, here we restrict his findings only to males, and in regard to three particular age groups, which we have tabulated as follows:

Age Group	Number	Per cent
40 to 49	373	28.7
50 to 59	498	38.2
60 to 69	267	21.0

You can see from this tabulation that the highest frequency fell in the age group from fifty to fifty-nine. The next highest fell, not in the following decade as would be expected, but in the preceding one. If age itself were a deciding factor, one would expect the incidence to be higher in those sixty to sixty-nine than in the group between forty and forty-nine. Yet the exact opposite is true.

This is not the only study that tends to contradict the theory of aging as the cause of heart attack. A recently published study carried out by a British physician shows that incidence of heart attack in men reached its highest peak between the ages of fifty-five and fifty-nine and thereafter fell sharply.

But perhaps the strongest evidence against the role of age is that the incidence among males is much greater than among females. If age were a factor, the same proportion of men and women in the same age group would come down with heart disease.

The evidence shows unmistakably that changes in the coronary do not come about because of the aging process itself. Yet the fact is that older persons are far more likely to suffer a heart attack than younger ones. How to reconcile this seeming contradiction?

The contradiction is only apparent, not real. A little consideration will show that the connection between age and heart attack is not a direct one.

Atherosclerosis and Age

Narrowing of the coronary does not necessarily mean that a person will suffer a heart attack. Far from it. *Only a rather small proportion of people with any degree of narrowing of the coronary will ever come down with a heart attack.*

Although you know your coronary must have been affected since you have had a heart attack, it by no means indicates that you will, of necessity, have another one. For this reason, you should have a clear understanding how and why a narrowed coronary artery may be perfectly compatible with good health.

You should keep in mind two well-established scientific facts. The first is that every person who is struck down with this type of heart attack has atherosclerosis of his coronary arteries.

The second and equally important one is that not everyone who has atherosclerosis will ever suffer a heart attack, even though he lives to the age of Methuselah.

These two propositions may seem at first contradictory. However, there is no contradiction implied at all. The first proposition is self-evident, but the second needs some elaboration.

There is practically no way today to tell the condition of the coronaries in the living person. Of course, if he has suffered a heart attack, we know definitely from that fact that his coronaries must have been affected. But if a person is apparently in good health, no method available at the present time, not even electrocardiogram, can reveal the condition of his coronaries.

The only way we can determine exactly what shape the coronaries are in is by examination after death. At autopsy, the pathologist examines the coronary, measures its diameter, and applies other highly accurate methods of analysis. Consequently, what we know about the prevalence of atherosclerosis among persons of various ages in the population is derived largely from the extensive reports of pathologists.

From such studies we know that at least a slight degree of narrowing of the coronary artery is present in most, but not all, persons who have passed the age of forty. But don't let that frighten you and, above all, don't imagine that just because you are forty or over you are a candidate for heart attack. Far from it.

In the first place, such slight narrowing in the lining of the coronary does not in the least interfere with its efficiency as a blood supply line. Experiments have shown that even a branch of the coronary artery narrowed to half its caliber for a stretch of almost an inch can deliver a sufficient amount of blood as efficiently as a normal artery. In the second place, the chances are excellent that this narrowing will never increase to such an extent as to affect the caliber to any significant degree.

But just how frequently does it happen that fatty deposit accumulates to such an extent that the coronary does become narrowed considerably?

In one large series of autopsies comprising 3,000 cases, pathologists found 1,629 of the hearts had coronaries that were significantly narrowed down at one point or more, despite the fact that many of these persons had died from some other causes.

In another series it was found that of all persons between thirty and thirty-nine who had died from other diseases, no less than 18 per cent had what was classified as severe scarring of the coronary at one place or other. In the same series, the majority of persons over forty-nine had a like grade of coronary artery narrowing. This may sound alarming, but such narrowing occurred in an extremely small branch of the coronary tree, the rest of it being perfectly normal.

From the fact that all these persons had died from something else, it is obvious that the narrowing of only a small branch does not necessarily affect the function of the heart. As a matter of fact, it is rare indeed to find the heart of a man or woman past the eighth decade of life that does not have at least minimal narrowing in some portion of the coronary tree. That they lived to a ripe old age should be definite proof that some narrowing of the coronary did not interfere with good health. Inversely, it has been stated that for a person to live to extreme old age he must have unusually good coronaries.

Even more to the point in proving that age alone does not account for deterioration of the coronary artery is the careful examination carried out by Dr. Paul Dudley White and his associates. They minutely examined the entire coronary tree of 600 men who had died from different diseases at the age of from thirty to eighty-nine. There were exactly 100 men in each of the six decades. They found that men between fifty and fifty-nine had the maximum degree of coronary narrowing. But they also found that the severity of narrowing was somewhat less in persons past the age of sixty, even though present to some degree.

It is true that the longer a person lives the longer the factors responsible for either atherosclerosis or heart attack itself can exert their adverse influence. In such an indirect way the factor of age can be said to play a role. But fundamentally, neither heart attack itself nor its underlying cause, fatty accumulation in the coronary artery, depends on age as such. So for a clue, or clues, we must look elsewhere.

Heart Attack in Men and Women

How often, when you have read of a prominent middle-aged person who died suddenly of a heart attack, was it a woman? Among your friends, relatives, and acquaintances who had a heart attack, how many were women? Some, but not many. Now and then you hear of a comparatively younger man in his thirties having a heart attack, but never a woman of that age. Of the 100 young coronary patients between twenty-two and forty in the Massachusetts Coronary Research Project, of which we shall have a good deal more to say, 97 were men and only three were women. This is representative of other studies of persons under forty, all of which include practically the same proportion of men to women.

Your impression, therefore, that men are infinitely more susceptible to heart attack than women is quite correct. Many aspects of coronary heart disease are still highly controversial, but no one disputes the fact that it is predominantly a disease of the male.

Why this enormous difference between the two sexes? After all, a man's heart functions exactly the same way as a woman's. In fact, except for the difference in primary and secondary sex characteristics, vital functions are exactly the same in women as in men. Yet there are often enormous differences between men and women in their susceptibility to various diseases, including coronary heart disease.

So far as coronary disease is concerned, the difference in incidence between men and women is particularly great in the younger age groups, a fact that may suggest a clue to why such a difference exists at all. In one study, the ratio under forty was found to be 9 to 1. Thereafter, the difference gradually decreases. Selecting a number of representative series, the ratio between men and women in various age groups is as follows:

	Ratio of
Age Group	*Men to Women*
Under 40	9 to 1
40 to 49	4 to 1
50 to 59	3 to 1
60 to 69	2 to 1
Over 70	Equal

Since these differences are so great and persist up to the age of seventy, there must be some explanation for them. The real question should not be why are men more susceptible to heart attack but, rather, why do women seem to be more protected against it?

There have been a number of theories advanced by way of explanation, but so far there is not a single one that is completely satisfactory. It may be, perhaps, that several factors together play a role in it. Or, as is more likely, there may be a central factor out of which all others arise.

One such theory claims that in women the body is better able to take care of the fatty substances circulating in the blood. Another theory is that women do less muscular work, so that the heart needs to pump less blood at each beat and, consequently, does not have to work so hard. Others have suggested that the periodic loss of blood through menstruation may ease the work of the heart, or perhaps that the dilatation of the small blood vessels of the womb at each period may similarly affect the other blood vessels of the body. It is hardly conceivable that such temporary and insignificant changes are sufficient to account for such striking differences.

The supposed difference in the amount of muscular work is certainly not true. In the first place, the difference in physical activity of men and women is not nearly so great as most people think. True, women do not perform heavy manual labor, but a glance at the table in Chapter 8 listing the energy requirements of ordinary household activities, or at the chart in Chapter 11 showing the comparison of energy used in daily life, proves that women do, indeed, perform a considerable amount of physical work. The busy housewife probably expends a good deal more energy in physical activity than most husbands do at their jobs.

Futhermore, the stress and strain connected with pregnancy and childbirth involves an extremely great and sudden increase in the demands of the heart, for which there is certainly no comparable strain for men.

At any rate, even if the physical work of the woman is, on the whole, less than that of the man, such a difference is not sufficient to explain the extraordinarily great difference in the incidence of heart attack.

Besides, why do women past fifty or sixty approach a closer level with men in incidence? To explain this difference on the basis of amount of physical work performed, one would have to presume that older women now work just as hard as men of the same age, which, of course, is an absurdity.

The Factor of Estrogen

During the first few years of research directed toward the solution of the problem of sex difference in heart attack, most investigators suspected that the female hormone, estrogen, had something to do with it. Then, unaccountably, the theory of estrogen as the real reason for the seeming protection of the female sex against heart attack somewhat lost favor among scientists. Yet considering all the facts, it is impossible to escape the conclusion that it is estrogen that accounts for this difference. Even though at present we do not know in what way estrogen performs this useful task, in the absence of any evidence to the contrary there is nothing that can more satisfactorily explain the enormous difference between incidence of heart attack in the two sexes.

Although the difference is not so great in regard to changes in the coronary artery itself as it is in heart attack, such changes past the age of forty are more severe in men than in women, probably because in men they begin earlier in life. That fact, again, points to the probable role of estrogen.

Perhaps the most striking evidence of the protective role of estrogen is that in women who have had both ovaries removed the incidence of heart attack is just about the same as in males of the same age. Removal of the ovaries, of course, means that no more estrogen will be produced, or if at all, then in a greatly diminished amount. That is exactly what happens in women past change of life. The ovaries cease to function and, therefore, no longer produce estrogen. This fact in itself is highly suggestive of why the ratio decreases considerably with advancing years until the age of seventy, when both men and women are equally susceptible to heart attack.

Some investigators objected to the estrogen theory because the incidence does not rise immediately after change of life. This is exactly what could be expected. It takes a long time, certainly years, until the accumulation of fatty deposit in the coronary artery affects its caliber to an appreciable extent. Now, if fatty substance begins to accumulate after change of life, it would take many years before it would interfere with coronary circulation and induce a heart attack.

That estrogen does have a protective value for the arteries, at least in animals, has been demonstrated by laboratory experiments. Hens are not subject to hardening of the arteries. However, after the ovaries are removed, they develop hardening of the arteries just as readily as cocks.

Other scientists lean to the theory of structural differences in the coronary arteries of the two sexes. There is definite evidence that a structural difference exists in the coronaries of males and females even at birth. Dr. W. Dock measured accurately the coronary arteries of a number of newborn infants of both sexes who had died shortly after birth. He found that the lining of the coronaries in the male infants was more than three times as thick as that in female infants. Other investigators later confirmed his findings. Dr. Dock believes that this greater thickness is sufficient to account for the striking difference in the incidence of heart attack in later life.

This advantage of females over males is not confined to coronary heart disease. So far as life expectancy is concerned, the female of the species has a decided advantage over the male. But it is also evident that the modern male is steadily adding to his native handicap. The death rate since the turn of this century has been steadily declining, but this decline is far greater for females than for males. The result, as could be expected, is that women finally caught up with men numerically, and are steadily increasing in number over males.

In 1945, for the first time in the history of the nation, women began to outnumber men in the total population. In the 1950 census the excess of females over males amounted to one per cent. By 1975, according to the calculation of the Metropolitan Life Insurance Company, this excess will amount to four per cent. No wonder public health officials began to speak of man as the "fragile male."

Here we are concerned only with the ever-increasing preponderance of females over males insofar as it is due to greater mortality from coronary heart disease in men. The latest vital statistical data are those for the year 1955. These figures show that 200,000 more males than females died in that year. Very nearly half of this excess was due to death from coronary heart disease. In round numbers 93,000 more males than females died in that year from coronary heart disease.

The reasons for the widening of this gap are many and varied. Its very existence, however, suggests that, in general, men may have adapted themselves less well to the stresses, tensions, and demands of modern life. Again, strange as it may sound at first, women may handle emotional problems more successfully than men. Dr. James Bond of the Florida State Board of Health expressed this very neatly when he said: "The wife may release her tensions through tears, while her husband must act manly and choke his back into his coronary arteries."

Decline of Physical Effort

However, the most important factor may be the abandonment of physical activity by modern men. Men are by nature dynamic.

Their heart seems to be attuned to the performance of muscular work, built in such a way as to require physical demands and challenges for its effective function. The highly mechanical nature of modern life, both at home and at the job, has brought with it labor-saving devices which, in turn, have led to corresponding decline in physical effort. This undoubtedly has its advantages. No one, least of all the medical profession, wishes a return to the back-breaking labor of the tens of thousands of slaves who built by brawn alone the magnificent pyramids of Egypt.

But sex is not the only characteristic that plays a role in relative susceptibility to heart attack. The tendency may also be inherited.

14

Heredity and Body Build

PHYSICIANS who have been in practice for some years occasionally have the experience of treating both a father and, years later, his son for a heart attack. In such instances, not infrequently both father and son are stricken with the disease at the same age.

The most notable of such cases is one in which the father suffered a heart attack at the age of forty-two. One of his sons was stricken when he was forty-three years old, another at the age of thirty, and the youngest at thirty-one.

These occurrences are not simply a matter of coincidence. It has been known for some time that there are certain families in which several members develop coronary disease. Evidence has been gathered that shows conclusively that it may run in some families.

The Role of Heredity

That heredity plays a definite role in coronary heart disease, no one doubts any more. But there is ample evidence that it is not the only role. The great majority of patients come from families none of whose members, so far as can be determined, have or had any kind of heart disease. Just because you come from a family with a bad history in this regard does not mean that you will necessarily develop it. Even in families which, so to say, are overladen with coronary disease, the majority of the members will not come down with it.

Nevertheless, if you have a bad family history, it is imperative that you undergo periodic examination by a physician. There is some evidence that high cholesterol level in the blood may also be an inherited characteristic. If your cholesterol happens to be high, you'll need to go on a special low cholesterol diet and, in general, arrange your life in such a way as not to invite a heart attack. But if the physician finds nothing wrong with you after repeated examination, you will have saved yourself a lot of needless worry.

The best way of studying the manner of transmission of traits, both mental and physical, is by the accurate examination of identical twins. In order better to appreciate the data derived from such studies, we need mention that there are two kinds of twins, fraternal and identical. By some chance, instead of one female egg, as is usual, there might be two present and fertilized at the same time. In that event, the two babies that develop from the two fertilized eggs will be related only as brothers and sisters and will have inherited characteristics present in the two fertilized eggs. These are fraternal twins.

The other type of twins develops from a single female egg, fertilized by a single male sperm. But soon after fertilization this egg splits into two, and each develops into a fully mature baby. These are called identical twins. Since both inherit exactly the same characteristics present in that single fertilized egg, they will be in all respects alike as two peas.

A good deal of what we know about the laws of inheritance in human beings has been derived from the study of identical twins. Now, if one of a pair of identical twins happens to break a leg or get pneumonia, the other, naturally, will not experience the same mischance. But if a disease or tendency to some kind of condition is transmitted as a hereditary characteristic, both twins should be afflicted with exactly the same disorder.

A few years ago a remarkable case of a pair of identical twins was reported in which both of the brothers developed severe angina pectoris, one at the age of thirty-four, the other at thirty-eight. This shows that at least the tendency to coronary heart disease may be directly transmitted.

The best information, and the most accurately controlled, not only in regard to the role of heredity but also in respect to a number of other factors, is furnished by the study carried out a few years ago in the Massachusetts General Hospital.

The Relation of Heredity to Heart Disease

Some twenty years ago, Drs. Glendy, Levine and White published a paper in which they analyzed the differences in regard to a number of traits between one hundred cardiac patients under the age of forty and a group of healthy older persons. One of the things they noted was that the majority of the patients were husky, rather muscular, and thick set.

What was the significance of this finding? Was it simply a coincidence, or did body build have something to do with proneness to develop coronary heart disease?

Other physicians made the same observation. Then, many other studies appeared that compared coronary patients and healthy individuals in a number of different ways. Out of such studies emerged a number of facts that offered a clue toward the solution of the problem of why certain persons are apparently more prone to heart disease than others. On the basis of these findings, Dr. White and his associates organized a systematic study to look for an answer to the many factors involved in it.

The plan was to examine, in every possible aspect, one hundred persons who had suffered a heart attack under the age of forty, but who had completely recovered and who had no other complicating condition as, for instance, high blood pressure or diabetes. The reason the investigators selected people under forty was to prevent the factors of age or other complicating disease conditions from obscuring the basic characteristics for which they were searching.

Out of 250 prospective subjects, 100 persons were selected who met every one of these requirements. Ninety-seven of these were males and three were females. Then 146 healthy male subjects were chosen as a control group. To make the comparison even closer, 97 of these were selected so as to match exactly one male patient in the coronary group in age, height, weight, body build, racial origin, and occupation. In this way, then, it was possible to make more exact comparison between healthy and coronary individuals and to see in what respects the two groups differed.

The ages of these men ranged from twenty-two to forty. Each patient selected for the study was admitted to the Massachusetts General Hospital and was kept there for 24 to 72 hours. During this stay, among other things, the family history of each was obtained, and each was examined by specialists in the respective fields; electrocardiograms were taken; body measurements were made; blood chemistry studies were carried out; and many other pertinent facts obtained. The group of healthy persons selected as controls underwent exactly the same examinations, so that it was possible to compare the two groups in every respect.

After the voluminous data of both patients and controls accumulated during this intensive examination were collected, the research team subjected them to searching analysis and at the end of two years published their findings. These data furnished material in regard to sex, heredity, body build, athletic background, occupation, physiological and psychological data, dietary, hormonal, and, in general, biochemical aspects. The information derived from this thorough study served to put on a sound basis the clues unearthed prior to this work, and to give many answers to some of the most puzzling questions.

Here we are concerned with the answer this study gave to the possible role of inheritance. For this part of the study the investigators obtained the medical history of the parents, grandparents, brothers and sisters of all male patients. At the same time, a similar history was obtained of the 146 healthy persons who were used as a control group.

A number of fathers and mothers of both groups were dead at the time of the investigation. After the cause of death of the parents of both groups was tabulated, a highly significant fact emerged:

18.5 per cent of the fathers *of the control group* had died from coronary disease.

31.7 per cent of the fathers *of the coronary group* had died from coronary disease.

This shows definitely that a person whose father acquires coronary heart disease has twice as great a chance of developing the same disease as a person whose father does not have coronary disease.

There was no difference in the percentage of deaths of the mothers in these two groups. This means that the tendency evidently is not transmitted on the mother's side.

The role of inheritance was then examined from another angle. A number of brothers and sisters of both groups had died at the time the compilation was made. When the cause of death of these brothers and sisters was tabulated, it was found that 8.6 per cent of brothers and sisters of the coronary group had died from coronary disease. Only one per cent of brothers and sisters in the control group had died from coronary disease.

The difference shows that the tendency to the disease may be transmitted to more than one member of the family.

Nevertheless, it does not follow that every one of the offspring, or even the majority, coming from such family will inevitably be afflicted. On the contrary, detailed genealogical trees prepared for both groups revealed that there were extremely few families in the coronary group in which another member was also afflicted with the same disease.

From this and other similar studies it is apparent that coronary disease runs in some families. But it is equally evident that in only exceptional cases will more than one member of the family inherit the tendency. Furthermore, whatever the factor transmitted to the offspring responsible for the development of coronary heart disease, it is only one factor, and not the most important one. This is obvious from the fact that of 73 of the 100 patients in the Massachusetts study, neither parent had the same disease.

We need to search for other clues as to why some persons are more prone to coronary disease than others. One of these clues concerns the type of body build.

Body Build

Is there any connection between physique and proneness to coronary heart disease?

Although it was suspected that there is a connection, not enough accurate measurements as to body build had been made among coronary patients and healthy individuals to allow a valid conclusion. One of the prime purposes of the Massachusetts study was to find an answer to this question.

In order to find a valid answer, no less than twenty-four different measurements were made in every one of the subjects, both coronary and control, and from these a physical profile of each emerged.

We are prone to judge a person's general state of health from his appearance. A florid and heavy-set individual is thought of as a likely candidate for a stroke, or is at least suspected of having high blood pressure. A thin and emaciated-looking individual is believed to be in delicate health. In either case the judgment may be wrong. Nevertheless, there seems to be a definite connection between general body build and proneness to certain ailments.

But general impression is not a very accurate guide in judging a person's body type. The only way to classify persons according to body type is by accurate measurements. The information furnished by these measurements is the basis of that branch of science called physical anthropology.

Dr. W. H. Sheldon devised a method of describing the physical type to which each individual belongs. He recognized three components of every person's physical make-up. One component he called endomorphy; the second, mesomorphy; and the third, ectomorphy.

Don't let these forbidding terms deter you. By describing pure types of each of these components, you will have no difficulty in understanding what these terms mean in actuality.

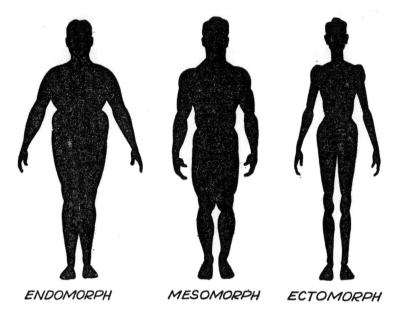

ENDOMORPH   MESOMORPH   ECTOMORPH

Figure 8. THE THREE BODY TYPES.

Endomorphy is the component of softness, roundness, and smoothness. A person who is predominantly endomorph is rounded in shape, and his anatomical features are "smooth." In such an individual, the angle between neck and chin is blunt, the chest is round, the thighs fit closely and he may be somewhat knock-kneed. He has small features and, in general, his measurements from back to front are greater than those from side to side.

The component of mesomorphy denotes muscularity, largeness of bones, and angularity. The person who is largely or predominantly mesomorph has large bones, the angle between neck and chin is rather sharp, his chest is deep, and he has powerful shoulders. His contour is tapering from shoulder to hips, he has heavy leg muscles, and broad hands and wrists. If the tips of your thumb and index finger do not touch when you put them around your wrist you have a mesomorph component in your body build.

Ectomorphy is a component of linearity, fragility, and tallness. An ectomorph has long fingers, long toes, long and narrow hands and feet. His chest is rather shallow, his waist is slender, and he has long legs. In general, he is a tall and lean individual. If the tips of your thumb and finger touch around your wrist, you have an ectomorph component in your make-up.

The real value of Sheldon's system is that he has given a numeric value to each of these three components present to varying degree in the make-up of every person. It will be sufficient to state that each component is given a number from 1 to 7, according to what extent it is present in a particular individual.

To give you an example, if a person is described in this system as endomorphy 7, mesomorphy 1, ectomorphy 2, it means that the person is predominantly endomorph, only to a slight degree mesomorph, and very little more ectomorph. Such a person, then, would be almost entirely a smooth and rounded individual, however with a few measurements that are slightly different. Or maybe another person rates as 2-6-2. That means he is predominantly mesomorph but not to an extreme degree, and that he has some features both endomorphic and ectomorphic.

Though no one is a pure endomorph, mesomorph, or ectomorph, a person is predominantly one or the other of these types.

When the body types of the coronary and healthy subjects were compared, it became evident that coronary heart disease was clearly associated with a definite body type. What was this specific type?

There was practically the same proportion in both groups of predominately endomorphs, the soft, round type.

There were only half as many predominantly ectomorphs, the tall, lean type, in the coronary group as in the control group.

There were twice as many dominantly mesomorphs, the husky, muscular type, in the coronary group as in the control group.

This study clearly demonstrated that the muscular, deep-chested, rather heavily built individual is the most prone to develop coronary heart disease. On the other hand, the lean, tall person with long hands and feet and rather shallow chest, is the least likely to develop coronary heart disease.

This does not mean at all that every coronary patient is of the mesomorph type, for there are many who do not correspond to it. And even more importantly, the overwhelming majority of persons with mesomorphic body build will never develop coronary heart disease. For *body build is only one factor* that may, but does not necessarily, predispose a person to it.

Nevertheless, this kind of body build is strikingly frequent among young coronary patients. What the significance of it is, no one knows. There are some clues that may, perhaps, offer some explanation. One of these is that many young coronary patients appear to be ten years older than their chronological age. Although not all physicians agree, some have noted that quite a number of their young coronary patients appear prematurely old. Dr. Milton Plotz states that 25 out of 30 coronary patients under the age of forty-five he has seen recently were noticeably bald or gray-haired.

Now, an older appearance is one of the striking characteristics of mesomorphs generally. Their skin is usually rather coarse and heavily wrinkled. Furthermore, mesomorphs usually reach the age of adolescence one to one and a half years earlier than boys of other bodily configurations, so that the reason they seem older than others of their age may be because they reach maturity earlier. Apparently, premature aging is due to the fact that they are mesomorphs, and not because they have coronary heart disease. On the other hand, it has been suggested that persons with predisposition for coronary changes also have a temperamental make-up conducive to faster living, which may account for apparently faster aging.

Quite a number of coronary patients seem to be hard-driving

and generally ambitious individuals, and have certain other temperamental characteristics in common. These same general characteristics are found among all mesomorphs. So, again, these traits may be due to body type and not to coronary disease itself.

It appears that what the individual does with his inborn equipment, how he lives, and particularly how much physical activity he maintains in advancing years may determine to a large extent how his coronaries stand up to various stresses and strains.

15

Physical Activity

A FEW years ago, Dr. J. N. Morris published a study that analyzed the incidence of coronary heart disease among the 25,000 employees of the London Transport Executive. The figures showed that the rate of heart attack was twice as great among the bus drivers as among the conductors of the same buses in comparable age brackets. To make sure it was not a chance occurrence, Dr. Morris repeated the analysis for the next two years. The results were exactly the same.

What could be the possible explanation of such striking difference? Bus drivers and conductors have the same social background and, in general, their living conditions are highly similar. Yet in at least one respect there is a good deal of difference between drivers and conductors. London buses are two-deckers, so that the conductor has to walk up and down a good deal, and is on his feet practically all the time during an eight-hour working day. The driver, during the same period of time, is glued to his seat and seldom has an opportunity to move about. In this case at least, the amount of physical work must have had something to do with it.

Dr. Morris and his co-workers then extended the study to a number of other occupations outside the transit workers so as to include postoffice employees, farmers, laborers, and a number of professional groups, covering altogether some

31,000 individuals. The results were startling. It became evident, for instance, that among postoffice employees a telephone operator has twice as great a chance of suffering a heart attack as a mail carrier of the same age. The postoffice telephone operator sits at his desk during the entire working day, while the postman walks or cycles and carries a good deal of mail.

In other kinds of occupations, similar difference was shown to exist. The incidence, again, was lower in those whose occupation involved a good deal of physical work, and practically proportional to the amount of physical work they performed.

From such observations, Dr. Morris came to the conclusion that the amount of physical work has a definite protective value against acquiring the disease. Or to put it conversely, lack of exercise and a sedentary mode of life predispose a person to it. The implication of this, if it could be proved for the general population and for all kinds of occupations, would be of tremendous practical importance. It would serve as a warning for a middle-aged person not to give up physical activity and adopt a wholly sedentary way of life and, thus, increase his chances of becoming a victim of heart attack. But it is even more important as a warning for anyone who has recovered from a heart attack. Slowing down too much and avoiding all physical activity can easily aggravate the condition.

What is the evidence that points to a definite connection between work and coronary heart disease? The evidence must of necessity be largely of a statistical nature. If two similar groups of persons differ considerably in the amount of physical work involved at their job and also in the rate of incidence of coronary disease, it would suggest that physical activity has at least something to do with it.

The Morris Studies

From the data of Dr. Morris, the death rate from coronary heart disease for various occupational groups at the same age levels can be calculated. For this we need to examine only the death rates of men in the forty-five to sixty-four age groups.

Out of each million hairdressers, for example, 880 die every year from this cause. At the other end of the scale are gardeners and laborers, for whom the death rate per million is only 150. The difference is tremendous. It is obvious that hairdressers do far less physical work than gardeners or laborers. But in between these two extremes, the death rate in different occupational groups varies from high to low, being, for example, twice as great among shoemakers as coal miners. It would obviously be impossible to grade with any exactitude the amount of physical work performed by various occupational groups. Nevertheless, it appears that, in general, the amount of physical work is in some way connected with the likelihood of developing heart attack.

Obviously we need some other kind of evidence. Such evidence is found in the mortality rates from coronary disease.

Dr. Morris and his co-workers examined the records of the Registrar General for the years 1930 to 1932. There it was shown that mortality was considerably lower among workers in occupations calling for heavy physical work than among those whose work was light.

In order to see whether the same conditions still prevailed at the time of the examinations, that is, twenty years later, the investigators examined the death certificates for every man between the ages of forty-five and seventy-four who had died from any cause in the two-week period during which the study was being carried out. The findings, again, were exactly the same as they had been twenty years before.

We need to mention only one more study, also carried out by Dr. Morris and his co-workers. They reviewed the autopsy records of workers in different types of jobs who had died from coronary disease. They found that the coronary arteries in men who had had lighter and less physically exacting jobs exhibited a much more severe form of coronary change than the arteries of men who had been employed in heavy work. They also found that for men whose occupations were classified as between these two extremes of physical activity, the severity of the coronary change was of a correspondingly intermediate nature.

From all this evidence Dr. Morris came to the conclusion that:

"Men in physically active jobs have a lower incidence of coronary heart disease in middle age than men in physically inactive jobs. The disease is not so severe in physically active workers, tending to be present in them first as angina pectoris and other relatively benign forms, and to have a smaller early case-fatality and lower early-mortality rate."

Dr. Paul Dudley White noted some time ago that: "One has the definite impression that it is distinctly less common in the lean laborer or farmer."

Occupational Hazards

Coronary disease has often been referred to as almost an occupational hazard of physicians. A good many studies have shown that, of all occupations or professions, it is particularly high, or perhaps the highest, among doctors. Specialists, such as gynecologists and surgeons, are even more vulnerable to it than are general practitioners.

The average specialist has largely an office practice, seldom goes on calls, and in general has more or less regular hours. On the other hand, the general practitioner has irregular hours, must make calls at all hours of the day and night, and altogether leads a far more active life. The latest national survey shows that the average family doctor spends about sixty hours a week in his work. Could it be, therefore, that the difference in physical activity accounts for the difference in incidence between specialists and general practitioners? It was not the conditions of the occupation, as such, that accounted for it.

Different occupations naturally involve different amounts of physical activity. In order to test the validity of the evident role of physical work, we must examine more closely the records of persons of various ages in various occupations. Again, the evidence is of a statistical nature. But these seemingly dry figures tell such a vivid story that it will be worthwhile to look at them, especially as two such statistics come from different parts of the world and from different time periods.

Some two decades ago a study appeared that tabulated all coronary deaths of white men in Philadelphia between the years 1933 and 1937, according to age and occupation. These men were divided into four occupational groups. The figures here refer to the annual death rate per 100,000 persons. In order to simplify the table, only the mean death rate for all men from thirty-four to sixty-four is listed.

Group	Death Rate per 100,00
Professional	154
Managers, etc.	140
Clerks, salesmen	128
Workers	107

It appears from this that the lighter the work involved, the greater the chances of dying from coronary.

Another study from another country and from a much later period tells the same story. This concerns the mortality rate from the disease of all men in England and Wales for the year 1951. The basis of comparison is different from that in the previous table, so an explanation will be necessary.

National statistics tell how many men die each year from the same disease, regardless of occupation. This number is taken as 100 per cent of the expected deaths from a particular disease for all the population. Now, when the death rate from coronary heart disease is computed for different categories of occupation, it is found that some occupational groups are either below or above this figure. For this purpose, the men were divided into five groups of occupation, and the ratio for each group was calculated, as shown in the table:

Group	Mortality Ratio
Professional	150
Farmers	110
Skilled workers	104
Unskilled workers	89
Partly skilled workers	79

You can now see that the mortality rate of professionals was 150, which means it is fifty per cent higher than the national average. But for partly skilled workers, such as mine workers, the ratio is considerably lower, that is, only seventy-nine per cent of the expected one.

All available evidence points unmistakably to the fact that sedentary life increases the chances of suffering a heart attack. But to what extent, and whether or not it does so invariably, has been seriously misunderstood by the general public.

When you read the statement of Dr. Morris that the incidence is twice as great among bus drivers as it is among bus conductors, you are likely to jump to the conclusion that everyone who has a more or less sedentary occupation is inevitably headed for a heart attack. To emphasize the beneficial effect of exercise in middle age is one thing. But to give the impression that all one has to do to avoid having a heart attack is to live a strenuous life is another thing altogether. One investigator believed that the reason so many middle-aged men of the country club kind suffer a heart attack is that they usually indulge in tennis, golf, or some other rather strenuous sport over the weekend but then fall back into completely sedentary habits for the rest of the week. Obviously, there are other factors than physical activity that might dispose a person to heart attack.

How over-generalization might be misleading could probably be illustrated by a no doubt far-fetched, but nevertheless applicable, example. Walking on an icy street on a bitter wintry day definitely has its hazards. A man may fall and break his leg. But this is entirely different from saying that he will invariably and of necessity do so. Of thousands and tens of thousands of people who walk on the busy streets of a large city, a few will actually fall, and one, or perhaps two, will break a leg. To say that icy streets are hazardous would be quite justified. But to say that the surest way to break a bone is to walk on an icy street would be a wholly unjustified over-statement. Dr. Morris himself put it this way: "A few will suffer it [coronary heart disease] and the great many do not."

The Rich and the Poor

One widely-held theory is that economic factors play an important role in predisposing to heart attack. Most people believe that coronary attack is particularly a disease of the rich. Some evidence seems, at first, to support this contention.

For example, when an investigator reviewed the autopsy records of some 3,400 persons who had died of various causes, he found that the incidence of rather severe deterioration of the coronary artery was twice as great among private patients as ward patients. From this it would seem that those who could afford to be attended by their own physician and, consequently, were in better economic circumstances and had lived a richer life, were particularly prone to it. But it may also be that the ward patients, exactly because of their lower economic status, had been engaged in work that involved mostly manual labor, while among the "rich" private patients there must have been a good many who had led a sedentary life.

This is only a speculation, not subject to exact proof. Nevertheless, we have some evidence that points to the amount of physical effort, not only in occupation, but also in the general way of life, as an important factor.

Sedentary vs. Active Life

There is still another way to look at the role of physical activity concerning greater susceptibility to heart attack. The work implied at the job is only part of the total physical exertion. How active a person is after quitting his desk or his machine may be quite as important.

It is often said that Americans have become largely spectators in sports events and participate very little in active sports; furthermore, that automobiles have eliminated a good deal of walking. In the last war a surprisingly large number of men were rejected by the Army because of lack of physical fitness. All this may be true to some extent but, on the whole, it seems an exaggeration. There is no actual evidence that the younger generation has become soft and flabby.

But in regard to middle-aged men, the story is different.

Most middle-aged men of the white-collar type have abandoned to a large extent any strenuous activity and, as a rule, have practically no physical hobbies or recreation. On the other hand, many workingmen of that age do participate a good deal in recreational activities such as bowling, fishing, and hunting.

You may be convinced by this time that sedentary life greatly increases the chances of coming down with a heart attack. But we can't say that lack of exercise initiates deterioration of the coronary artery. Of that we have no evidence. It would be difficult to imagine how slowing down in middle age could start fatty deposits in the lining of the coronary.

But there can no longer be any doubt that lack of activity aggravates a condition that is already present. You may say, of course, that you can't undo the damage already done by starting exercise now. But this is exactly what you should do. You remember we have stated that gradual and carefully graded physical activity favors the development of collateral circulation. Experiments have shown that, following artificial closing up of one branch of the coronary artery, animals subjected later to a good deal of exercise developed much more efficient collateral channels than animals kept at rest during the same period of time. But it is equally true that these collateral blood vessels that become enlarged following the plugging up of a main branch do not stay open indefinitely. If stimulation no longer is present, these channels, so to say, collapse and are no longer adequate. Now, the necessary stimulation that keeps these channels open and even further enlarges them is best furnished by physical activity. If the need for a supplemental supply of blood is constantly present, collateral circulation will continue and will even improve appreciably. Such need arises from the greater use of the heart.

Overweight

A sedentary life means more than simply lack of exercise. Middle-age spread is due in great part to the fact that the man who quits most of his physical effort puts on considerable weight because he no longer burns up the excess calories. This sets up a vicious circle, as the overweight person also tends to avoid all exertion.

Does serious overweight predispose a person to develop coronary artery deterioration? Frankly, there is no general agreement on this point among the best authorities. A number of studies show that there are a large number of obese persons in the coronary groups. Others doubt any connection between obesity and coronary disease.

One way to decide this question is to compare the percentage of obesity among persons who have suffered a heart attack and among healthy individuals of the same age and sex. A number of large-scale studies have been carried out to find an answer. The reported results, however, were conflicting. Yet it would be extremely important to find a clear-cut answer, since overweight is so prevalent in America today. In a recent study of 10,000 unselected persons, around 28 per cent were found to be 10 per cent or more above their ideal weight according to sex, age, and height.

Some studies have shown that a large proportion of patients suffering from coronary disease are overweight or obese according to the standard tables. A curious finding in many of these studies is that obesity appears to be connected with coronary heart disease in men but not in women. In other studies, however, investigators were unable to find any connection at all between overweight and coronary heart disease, in either men or women.

The best and most thorough study to find an answer to the possible role of overweight is the Massachusetts Coronary Research Project, to which we have referred so often. Dr. Gertler and his co-workers approached the problem from an entirely different angle. After reviewing the entire medical literature on the subject, they came to the conclusion that the usual standard weight tables can be highly misleading. These tables may show that a man is seriously overweight, yet that weight may be just right for him because he is large-boned and is of a particular body build. Any consideration of weight measurements must include the factors of age, sex, height, and body build.

The standards adopted by the U.S. Army fulfill these requirements. Using these Army standards, Dr. Gertler found that the coronary and the control groups do not differ at all in regard to overweight. At least in younger persons the matter of weight has no significance in predisposing to coronary heart disease.

But there is one thing about which there cannot possibly be any disagreement, and that is the importance of weight reduction for persons who have aready suffered a heart attack. Any person who is seriously overweight imposes a much greater load on his heart. His work tolerance is seriously impaired, and he evidently has less heart reserve to meet extra demands. A fat man or woman avoids all kinds of physical effort and activity.

The advice Dr. Wartenberg gave to his doctor friend in the letter we have mentioned before is very much to the point:

> You have to lose every single drop of superfluous fat. This is final. And no bargaining about you. You must be here extremely strict with yourself. Find out your normal weight and get it; by all means, under any circumstances. But lose slowly—one pound a week is enough.

It is not only the energy expended in physical activity, however, that has a direct effect on the proper function of the heart. Emotions and mental work also cost a good deal of energy. Here the question is not how much energy the brain uses up but, rather, to what purpose it is used. In other words, we need to examine to what extent emotions, temperament, and tensions may predispose a person to heart attack.

16

Temperament and Tension

WE ARE constantly told that the terrible strains and stresses of life today create so much anxiety, tension, and restlessness that an ever-increasing number of people pay for them in peptic ulcer, asthma, or colitis, all diseases in which emotional disturbances play a prominent role. The complexities, the almost unbearable tempo, and the competitive urge of industrial society are blamed for the prevalence of the modern scourge: coronary heart disease.

In contrast, life in the past is pictured as one of comparative simplicity, tranquility, and leisure, singularly free of all the disturbing complications with which we have to contend today. You have probably read a period novel of the Victorian age in which the whole family leads a sheltered life, the father does not have to gulp down his breakfast so that he can catch the local train, the son does not seek excitement by driving all over the countryside at breakneck speed in Dad's high-powered car, the daughters stay home to help Mamma in her household duties, the menial tasks are performed by maids, cooks, man-servants. The picture no doubt evoked an almost envious nostalgia in you. The "olden times," you would say, were certainly immensely different from conditions of the present.

Past and Present

But throughout the ages, "olden times," the past, has always appeared in shining colors to each new generation. It is often amusing to read the commentaries of contemporaries of any age, maybe many centuries ago, who speak of their own grandfathers' time as old-fashioned, simple, and uncompli- cated compared to the life of their own generation, which they think of as hard, difficult, and complex. They speak of the times they live in as the most trying in all history, replete with problems mankind was never confronted with before. Does not that sound a little like the way we speak of our own times? Has there ever been, except in retrospect, an undisturbed, serene, and idyllic period in the history of mankind? Is the age in which we are living so soul-trying, so difficult, so unimaginably strenuous as to make it nearly beyond the ability of any man to achieve even a semblance of success without utter havoc to his emotions?

But where is the proof that our ancestors were not subjected to just as much stress, anxiety, worry, fear, insecurity as the people of our own generation? Surely they must have faced exactly the same personal and interpersonal problems, just as painful, imminently hopeless, and devastating, as we do. A young man of a hundred and fifty years ago, hopelessly and desperately in love with a young damsel, suffered agonies just as acute as a young man of today does. Look at some of the charming pictures of days long gone by, with little tots gamboling and frisking just as children do today. Men and women were constituted exactly alike in all ages, and con- sequently responded in exactly the same way and to the same degree to immediate situations as do men and women today.

Were men of the past less capable of meeting the challenges of civilization? If it were possible, as in science-fiction, to resurrect a gentleman of the era of the American Revolution and place him in the middle of a busy street in New York, he would unquestionably be bewildered and lost. But not for long. Being a human being, exactly as we are, he would soon adjust himself to skyscrapers, buses, planes, elevators, and to all the conveniences of modern life.

How can anyone prove that our age is more troubled and stressful than any other period in history? As a matter of fact, a good case could be made out for exactly the opposite by selecting facts according to what we would be trying to prove.

The westward migrants were faced with daily dangers in their trek into unconquered and hostile wilderness, as well as from no less hostile Indians, and had to hew out new homes and wrest a livelihood while faced with the ever-present menace of starvation. Surely they must have experienced as much stress in their daily lives as their descendants who live under much more settled conditions and who, at least, no longer have to fight with hostile nature.

If stress alone could be blamed for deterioration of the coronary and subsequent heart attack, the rate of heart attacks should have increased tremendously during the occupation of Norway in the war days. Yet exactly the opposite occurred. There was a decline in the rate of as much as 20 to 25 per cent during the period in the general population of Norway. Some investigators attributed this striking decrease to the severe restriction of fat in the daily diet during the war. Yet the fact is that a decline in incidence began even before the war years.

Stress and Personality

The fact is that tensions, stresses, emotional burdens, the inner difficulties, the intimate personal problems, are the same in every age and do not depend on the contrivances and external trappings of any civilization. It is the internal milieu of every man and woman that determines how he reacts to any problem. Any problem has significance only when it arises, and then only in a strictly personal sense. As one thoughtful physician expressed it: "No one can measure emotional stress, since it has no meaning except in relation to him who is stressed."

Emotional stress, tension, and anxiety do not depend on external circumstances in which the individual finds himself, but on his ability to handle stressful situations. A phlegmatic type of person, not easily excitable, one who faces situations with equanimity, will react to conditions of living in exactly the same way regardless of the period in history in which he happens to be born. An anxious, fearful, uncertain and insecure individual will be greatly disturbed by conditions and will react in an exaggerated manner to external stimuli, even though he live during the most peaceful, secure, and undisturbed period in history.

But what is stress after all? You have been told so often that you must avoid frustrations, anxiety, grief, tension, and in general any stressful situation, whatever that is. You are warned not to give free play to emotions of any kind lest it injure your heart. In the same breath and with equal plausibility, you are told that repression of hidden desires will surely lead to inner conflict and anxiety, the source of neurotic symptoms. Which advice should you follow?

Emotional stress has acquired such a bad reputation that we have come to believe the ideal life one in which no stressful situation could possibly arise. Yet such a vegetative and overly placid life is not only wholly unattainable, but if it could be achieved might prove harmful. Joy, pride, striving, and attempts at the solution of life's problems also involve emotional stress. If one eliminates completely the supposedly bad emotional stresses and tensions, life itself would also be limited. And no one has yet proved that stressful situations compatible with "normal" life will ever lead to deposits of fatty substances in the coronary artery.

Even if emotional turmoils are extremely high they do not necessarily produce greater susceptibility to coronary heart disease. The incidence of coronary disease is no greater among psychiatric patients with manic-depressive disease, which is certainly productive of extreme emotional swings, than it is among the general population. Nevertheless, there are many persons who react to stress of any kind in an exaggerated manner. Can such exaggerated reaction damage the coronary arteries?

It may be that in such persons this inner turmoil flows back, so to say, to the coronary arteries. How such excessive emotional influence could be reflected in bodily organs in susceptible individuals has been variously explained. It has been claimed that emotional stimuli can increase the tendency of the blood to clot. Naturally, in persons who already have a great accumulation of fatty substances in the lining of their coronaries, this increased ability of the blood to clot may conceivably precipitate formation of thrombus. Fear, anxiety, sudden fright, as is well known, instantly mobilize the defense mechanisms of the body. This defensive reaction involves a sudden increase in and flooding of the blood with adrenalin, a hormone produced by glands situated atop the kidneys. Adrenalin has the effect of shortening the clotting time of the blood, so that it is easily conceivable that it may lead to formation, or at least easier formation, of thrombus in the coronary artery.

We also have evidence that emotional stress may increase the cholesterol content of the blood, and also may produce increase in the fatty deposit in the coronary arteries. It is known, too, that fear can produce significant changes in an electrocardiogram. Again, steady impact of nerve impulses may affect the tone of the coronary artery.

Whatever the mechanism, it seems certain that emotional factors may increase the chances for a heart attack in susceptible individuals. However, there is no way of telling who these individuals are. It seems to depend a good deal on the personality pattern.

Personality Pattern and Coronary Disease

The question of the greater proneness of some people to suffer heart attack is one of the most controversial in the whole field of coronary heart disease. Some authorities claim that one could predict who is likely to suffer a heart attack from evaluation of his emotional traits. Other scientists who have pursued the subject just as thoroughly deny the existence altogether of specifically heart-attack-prone individuals. The debate is far from being resolved one way or the other, at least in any way convincing enough to allow one to take a definite stand on it. Dr. Paul Dudley White states that medical science should be concerned not so much with the disease itself as with "the person who develops heart disease."

More than two decades ago, Dr. H. F. Dunbar, in an authoritative work, *Emotions and Bodily Changes,* studied the personality pattern of a number of coronary patients. She found that these patients had an unusually high rate of previous ailments. Their rate of marriages was high, and many of them had large families. Most of them had completed whatever educational courses they had undertaken. Significantly, many of them had continued at the same job for long periods of time, worked long hours, and were rather reluctant to take vacations.

Few of them had any interest in sports or hobbies but preferred to follow intellectual pursuits. On the surface, these patients appeared to be unusually calm. However, when they were questioned more closely it was found that they had carried over into mature life inner conflicts that had arisen in childhood. According to Dr. Dunbar, most of them had been rather stubborn, self-willed, and given to brooding when they were children. Psychoanalytic probing showed that many of them had had an early competitive relationship, usually with the father, which led to a subconscious conflict that evidently had colored their entire lives. In adulthood, this competitive attitude was transferred to others in positions of authority. According to her statements, many of them had a compulsive nature, and yet hard work and self-discipline brought no personal gratification.

Other investigators stated that the personality pattern of coronary patients included a need for and respect of authority. They had a compulsive tendency, a feeling of insecurity and inferiority. They exhibited asceticism and expended a great deal of effort at self-control. Of course, one may object to such a description of a personality pattern as too general, and applicable as well to a large group of neurotics who have nothing wrong with their heart.

Later investigators, however, were unable to confirm the studies of Dr. Dunbar and others. Notable among these is Dr. H. H. W. Miles and his co-workers, who compared forty-six coronary patients with forty-nine controls. Although Dr. Miles denies the existence of a specific coronary personality, he, too, found some differences in traits in the two groups. Coronary patients were somewhat less introspective than healthy individuals, and they had greater difficulty in handling their aggressive tendencies.

"The coronary patients," Dr. Miles wrote, "had tended to work harder, under more stress and strain. . . . More of the coronary patients than controls showed a consistent tendency toward compulsive striving, ascetic self-discipline, and great need to 'get to the top' in their chosen work."

Recently, instead of searching for a specific behavior pattern, investigators approached the problem from a different angle. Without claiming that a particular life history can lead to coronary disease, they attempted to describe the common traits of the coronary man.

The "Coronary Man"

Dr. Stewart G. Wolf, Jr., Professor of Medicine of the University of Oklahoma, in a panel discussion held at a recent meeting of the American Heart Association, presented a word portrait of a "coronary man." Dr. Wolf claimed that coronary patients can be identified by certain personality traits. He did not say, of course, that everyone with such traits will invariably develop the disease. But what he claims is that coronary men have certain striking characteristics.

He compared the coronary man to King Sisyphus of Greek mythology who, to expiate his sins, was condemned by the gods after death to pass his time in Hades by pushing a large rock up a steep hill. He never succeeded in getting the rock quite to the top, and as it rolled back he had to start over and over again in his futile try. The coronary man, Dr. Wolf says, is always looking for a new world to conquer, derives no satisfaction from achievement, and has no time to rest between chores.

According to this view, the coronary man is highly competitive in his basic attitude, concerned with self-sufficiency. He wants to do things in his own way, and usually the hard way. Such persons respond to emotional influences in an unusual manner. Dr. Wolf found that following unusual stress every one of the coronary patients exhibited a rise in blood cholesterol level, despite the fact that their diet did not vary at all.

At the same panel discussion, Drs. Meyer Friedman and Ray H. Rosenman of San Francisco presented a study that strongly supported the probable influence of emotional factors in coronary heart disease. They examined three groups of men matched in height, weight, and age, all of whom were engaged in light physical work. The first group consisted of tense, hard-driving individuals. The second, of easy-going persons. In the third group were unemployed blind men, who, understandably, would be under certain stress, but whose personalities closely resembled those of the easy-going group. When they compared these three groups, they found that among the driving type the incidence of manifest heart disease was 28 per cent; in the other two groups it was only 4 per cent. Even more striking were the findings for actual heart attack: 8 per cent in the first group, and none in the other two.

Another study presented at the same panel discussion further supported the possible influence of emotional factors in coronary heart disease. Dr. Henry I. Russek reported the result of a study made in a Staten Island hospital which compared 100 coronary patients with an equal number of healthy persons of the same age. He found that 91 of the coronary group either held down two jobs or worked more than 60 hours a week, or had personality problems characterized by insecurity or frustration. Only 20 of the control group matched this description.

Yet other investigators do not agree with this view. Perhaps the emotional factors have been overemphasized, or, as Dr. I. H. Page recently stated, "Stress has been overstressed." At any rate, stress cannot be measured.

Nevertheless, the evidence that emotion does sometimes play an important role is too strong to be easily rejected. Perhaps we cannot pinpoint the personality factors that are at least capable of aggravating an already present coronary disease. For that we shall need much more extended studies in the area of psychology.

There are many well-documented cases in which a sudden heart attack has followed some great emotional shock or overwhelming grief. Dying from a broken heart was a well-known device of nineteenth-century fiction. The young heroine, sorely disappointed in love, of course always at the end of the novel, simply lies down and dies from a broken heart. Today, when readers are more sophisticated, novelists are wary of using this highly convenient way to end the story. Yet such tragic events do occur in real life, although hardly to young heroes or heroines.

It happens that an elderly husband, learning of his wife's death, dies of a heart attack. Sometimes we read of a middle-aged man who collapses and suffers a heart attack while watching an exciting baseball or football contest. Other instances of heart attack under great emotional stress are certainly not an extraordinary rarity.

The question naturally arises, why did that particular person in any of these circumstances suffer a sudden heart attack when there must have been many others with diseased coronaries who faced similar situations without suffering a heart attack? At the baseball or football game there must have been others who had equal degree of coronary disease and who were subjected to the same amount and degree of excitement, and yet who did not suffer a heart attack because of it. Might it not be that a person with a particular basic personality type would tend to respond to a stressful situation to a much greater degree than a person with a different type of basic personality?

But how can we judge a person's basic personality? Too often we confuse what a man's personality is with what he actually achieves in life. A hard-driving and ambitious man, despite his constant striving, may remain all his life in an inferior position. On the other hand, an easy-going person who is well-adjusted may, and often does, rise to the top. Nevertheless, when we read of a prominent man being stricken with a heart attack, we are too ready to jump to the conclusion that it was his relentless drive and the tremendous responsibility of his position that has, so to say, burned up his coronaries. As a matter of fact, most people believe that coronary disease is particularly a disease of the executive. But is it actually so?

The Executive

You remember that Dr. Morris in his study of London transport workers found that bus drivers have twice as great an incidence of coronary disease as do bus conductors. The drivers, he pointed out, are constantly confronted with the extremely congested London traffic and, therefore, are under considerably more stress with more responsibility than conductors presumably are. So at least in part, the emotional stress may contribute to this poorer showing so far as heart attack is concerned.

But it may not be responsibility in itself that produces emotional stress. Instead, it may perhaps be the ability to meet responsibility, or the emotional attitude assumed in the face of responsibility, that is more significant insofar as the likelihood of acquiring coronary heart disease is concerned. At least, this is what is indicated in a study published recently in the Journal of the American Medical Association. This study directly contradicts the popular belief that coronary disease is a disease of executives. Drs. R. E. Lee and R. F. Schneider made repeated examinations over a period of more than five years of all white-collar employees of a large company located in a metropolitan area. They divided the 2,373 employees of this company, all working in the same building, into two main groups: executives and non-executives. The executive group included members of the board of directors, corporate officers, general managers, heads of divisions and departments, auditors, in short, all who were policy-makers. These numbered 1,171, all of whom were males. The non-executives numbered 1,202, of whom 563 were females, and included stenographers, secretaries, clerks, assistant supervisors, and supervisors.

The investigators restricted their studies to the male employees over forty years of age. They found that in these employees the incidence of coronary disease and heart attack was disproportionately lower among executives than among non-executives. The incidence was almost twice as great in the non-executive group.

Trying to explain such a surprising and wholly unexpected finding will naturally raise as many new questions as it will answer. Nevertheless, there are some possibilities that appear reasonable. It may be that persons who attain high positions are, to begin with, in exceptionally good health, so that they are able to absorb the greater demands on their emotions without impairing their general health. That these persons are usually in much better financial situation and can afford better medical care is certainly not valid for this group, for the organization offers a high-grade medical service regardless of the person's position in the company. It could be, of course, as these investigators suggest, that executives have a better education and better training, and so have learned the value of escape valves and "the need for outside avenues of expression, such as hobbies."

It may also be that the executive intrinsically worries less about his adequacy for the job, for his very position is a testimony that his ability has already been recognized. Thus, he will feel a good deal more self-confidence for the task with which he is confronted. These investigators also suggest that it is not the stress of the job itself that is significant, but rather the individual response to stressful situations. This again strongly supports the view we expressed before that it is not the nature of the stress but the nature of the man that counts.

If no study, no matter how detailed, has ever been able to pinpoint a single factor that predisposes a person to heart attack, the inevitable conclusion must be that no single factor exists. Heart attack is, so to say, the end result of a lifetime of living, and, at that, a lifetime of living by such an enormously complex biological unit as man. What can be more natural than to suppose that the end result, that is, heart attack, should arise from the gradual breakdown of many, perhaps innumerable and highly correlated, functions of the whole body? These individual factors may cancel out or counteract others.

All we can state is that there are harmful influences, some fairly well established and others only suspected, that, to say the least, certainly can do no good. However, to say—and many do, without factual basis—that these conditions are inevitably harmful for the individual is to go beyond the evidence we now possess. A hard-driving, ambitious man, overwhelmed with personal and interpersonal problems, may take a good deal of punishment without damage to his coronary system. But it is usually such a hard-driving type of individual who, if he does have a heart attack, is likely to become completely disorganized. For the calmer, more easy-going man, who is emotionally better adjusted and who does not overestimate his position in the scheme of things, heart attack is usually less disastrous insofar as his emotional reaction is concerned. For the more vigorous and impatient man, it may come as a shock, and he may collapse so completely that he swings to the other extreme and becomes an emotional invalid.

We have some evidence that strongly suggests the way the person reacts to his illness may have far-reaching psychological consequences. And such evidence is furnished by the masculinity tests carried out in the Massachusetts Coronary Research Project.

Masculinity—Physical and Psychological

In this study, the investigators examined the masculine traits, physical and psychological, in both the coronary and the control groups. In order to determine how the two groups compare in regard to the physical aspect of masculinity, they made a good many measurements, such as the amount and distribution of body hair, contour, assays of male hormones, and many others. They found that the typical coronary patient is much more masculine in physical aspect than the average control subject.

The investigators then turned to evaluation of the psychological aspect of masculinity. We need not go into detailed description of how masculine and feminine psychological traits are distinguished. It will be sufficient to state that some time ago psychologists devised a sort of IQ test by which a rating of psychological differences between male and female traits can be made. For instance, emotional responses differ for men and women. Women are more likely to express disgust at repugnant habits of dress and person, coarse language, and sexual immorality. Again, women express more liking for working with men than men do for working with women.

Word association will usually be different. Given a word, women usually associate it with terms for domestic things, while men are more likely to choose scientific or business terms. These tests, of course, included a good many other response patterns. Whatever the shortcomings or objections may be to this method of determining masculinity or femininity, the scoring from consideration of all responses together can be taken as reliable.

When the investigators evaluated the psychological components of masculinity it was found, surprisingly, that the coronary patients showed more reaction patterns that are typically feminine than the control group. The coronaries, as a group, were somewhat less aggressive, adventurous, enterprising, and less self-assertive, all of which are typically feminine traits.

How to reconcile this contradiction—prominent physical masculinity and more or less feminine psychological reaction?

A probable explanation is that a high component of physical masculinity had been tempered or modified by the illness itself. An originally hard-driving individual, determined to succeed and engaged in vigorous activity, may have become more introspective with a subsequent turning toward more cultural interests.

Whatever the explanation, it seems certain that the cumulative effect of inner tension in those particularly susceptible can be extremely powerful.

A Full Life

As we have seen, emotional upheaval is even more likely to provoke anginal attack than is overexertion. The same is equally true of any degree of coronary heart disease. But how to avoid stresses and tensions is another matter.

It is never easy to change a lifelong habit and an ingrained pattern of response. Nevertheless, mental discipline, retraining of the mind as well as the muscles, can succeed to a great degree. But if you go at it as a task and, even more importantly, if you look at it as a sacrifice, a concession to your ailment, you may actually aggravate your condition. The aim should be to live as full and normal a life as possible. And you can achieve this by economizing on your mental and emotional, as well as physical, expenditures.

If you put things in proper perspective, you will find that a good many things you have been doing and the way you have been doing them have been wholly unnecessary. Such a seemingly unimportant habit as carrying over your business worries to your home and planning the next day's schedule can create an atmosphere of tension and so prevent you from relaxing completely. A British physician found that when sleep is disturbed by exciting dreams the blood pressure rises considerably. Other investigators by accurate measurements found that emotional tension, besides raising the blood pressure, increases the pulse rate and raises the output of the heart, all of which, of course, places extra burden on the work it has to do.

But it is equally true that being constantly preoccupied with the condition of the heart will easily cause marked anxiety, which, in turn, leads to a state of semi-invalidism. Of course, it is not easy to strike a proper balance between recognizing the need of economizing on emotional expenditure and leading as active a life as possible. Moderation, however vague and trite it may sound, is the key word.

In the final analysis, moderation is dictated by common sense. It means a good deal more than avoiding strenuous work, cutting down on fats and calories in general. It also means that you should avoid situations that create emotional tensions and cut down on needless and tiresome social life. After all, at your age, a comparatively quiet life will give you far more inner satisfaction than trying to set the world on fire.

Above all, you should not think you are living on borrowed time. After you have recovered from a heart attack, your new life may be as full and content as though it had never been interrupted by that episode. Ultimately, it will be up to you. The best heart specialists, who have seen many thousands of cases over the years, are today highly optimistic about the outlook for a useful and productive life after heart attack. There is every reason that you, too, should be optimistic. You can live a full life after a heart attack.

Glossary

ANEMIC—lacking in either quantity or quality of blood.

ANEMIC HEART MUSCLE—temporary deprivation of blood of a tiny portion of the heart muscle.

ANGINA PECTORIS—periodic attacks of pain and of feeling of oppression under the breast bone, especially after exertion or emotional upset, usually due to diseased condition of the coronary artery.

ANTICOAGULANTS—drugs to prevent clotting of the blood.

AORTA—the largest artery of the body, originating from the heart.

ARTERIOLES—the smallest branches of the arteries.

ARTERIOSCLEROSIS—hardening of the arteries.

ARTERY—blood vessel carrying blood from the heart to all parts of the body.

ATHEROMA—fatty deposit in the lining of an artery.

ATHEROMATOUS PATCHES—spots of fatty deposits in the lining of an artery.

ATHEROSCLEROSIS—a form of hardening of the arteries characterized by fatty deposits in the lining of the artery.

AUSCULTATION—listening to the sounds produced by heart or lungs, by means of a stethoscope.

CAPILLARIES—minute blood vessels connecting the smallest branches of the arteries with the smallest branches of the veins.

CARDIAC RESERVE—ability of the heart to respond to extra demands placed upon it.

CARDIOPHOBIAC—person with a perfectly normal heart who is obsessed with the idea he has heart trouble.

CHOLESTEROL—a fatty substance circulating in the blood.

COLLATERAL CIRCULATION—small blood vessels that supply blood to an area deprived of blood because of closure of the main branch.

CORONARY—popular term for "coronary artery."

CORONARY ARTERY—artery of the heart itself.

CORONARY INSUFFICIENCY—inability of the coronary artery to supply enough blood for suddenly increased demands.

CYANOTIC—term used to describe blueness of the face caused by lack of sufficient oxygen in the blood.

DICUMAROL—a drug that prevents clotting of the blood; one of the most widely used anticoagulants.

DYSPNEA—difficulty in breathing.

ECTOMORPH—an individual with a shallow chest, long hands, feet, and legs, usually tall and fragile.

ELECTROCARDIOGRAM—record on scaled paper of electrical impulses produced by the action of the heart, used in diagnosis and also to check progress after heart attack.

ENDOMORPH—soft, rounded, smoothly built individual, prone to become obese.

H. A.; HEMORRHAGIC AGENT—any substance that can cause excessive bleeding.

HEPARIN—drug that retards or prevents clotting of the blood; one of the anticoagulants, made from the extract of ox liver.

INFARCT—portion of tissue suddenly deprived of its blood supply by a thrombus; it is replaced by scar tissue.

INTIMA—inner layer of all arteries, including the coronary.

INTRAVENOUSLY—injecting medication directly into the vein by means of a needle and syringe.

MEDIA—the middle layer of an artery.

MESOMORPH—muscular, robust and husky individual with deep chest, heavy legs, broad hands; particularly prone to develop heart attack.

MURMUR—blowing or hissing sound heard by the physician in listening to the heart, usually but not always indicating defect in a heart valve.

MYOCARDIAL INFARCT—the tiny portion of the heart muscle that dies out when the branch of the coronary that furnishes blood for it is plugged up; later transformed into a scar.

OCCLUSION—plugging up of one branch of the coronary artery.

PERICARDIAC SAC—a thin membrane that encloses the heart like a plastic bag.

RECANALIZATION—reopening of the channel in the coronary artery so the blood can flow through it again after the blood clot in it has been absorbed.

SATURATED FAT—fat that is solid at room temperature; of animal origin, with the exception of fish, the fat of which is unsaturated.

SEDIMENTATION TEST—a laboratory test to determine the speed with which red blood cells sink to the bottom of a test tube; a faster than normal rate indicates possible heart attack.

SUBCUTANEOUS—literally, under the skin; term used for injecting drugs under the skin.

SUBSTERNAL—under the breast bone; medical term used to distinguish pain that is felt under the breast bone from pain around the heart.

THROMBOSIS—the process of formation of a blood clot inside an artery.

THROMBUS—the blood clot itself inside an artery.

TRANSAMINASE—chemical substance present in normal heart muscle.

TRANSAMINASE TEST—special laboratory test to determine the exact amount of transaminase in the blood; increase usually indicates some damage to the heart muscle.

UNSATURATED FAT—fat that is liquid at room temperature, usually of vegetable origin, but also characteristic of fat from fish; can be transformed into saturated fat by manufacturing processes, as, for instance, in margarine.

VASOCONSTRICTION—temporary narrowing of the caliber of the arteries by muscular contraction of their wall.

VEINS—blood vessels that carry used blood back to the heart from all parts of the body.

Index

204